THE
English Physician

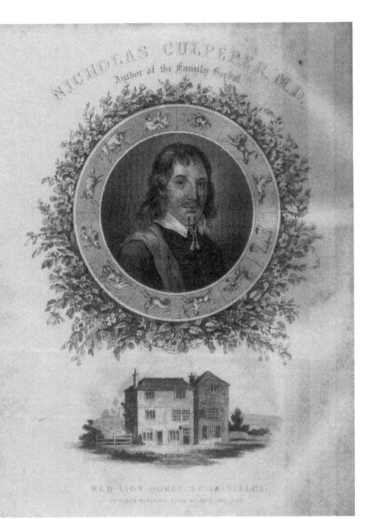

NICHOLAS CULPEPER, M.D.

Author of the Family Herbal

RED LION HOUSE, SPITALFIELDS.

THE
English Physician

NICHOLAS CULPEPER

Edited and with an introduction by MICHAEL A. FLANNERY

The University of Alabama Press

Tuscaloosa

The University of Alabama Press
Tuscaloosa, Alabama 35487-0380 uapress.ua.edu

Hardcover edition published 2007.
Paperback edition published 2014.

Inquiries about reproducing material from this work should be addressed to
the University of Alabama Press.

Typeface: AGaramond
Manufactured in the United States of America
Cover illustration: From *The Complete Herbal* (London: Thomas Kelly, c. 1830).
Reynolds Historical Library, University of Alabama at Birmingham
Cover design: Michele Myatt Quinn

∞

The paper on which this book is printed meets the minimum requirements of
American National Standard for Information Science–Permanence of Paper for
Printed Library Materials, ANSI Z39.48-1984.
    The information contained in *The English Physician* should in no way be
construed as practical, modern medical advice.
Paperback ISBN: 978-0-8173-5802-0

A previous edition of this book has been catalogued by the Library of Congress
as follows:
    Library of Congress Cataloging-in-Publication Data
    Culpeper, Nicholas, 1616–1654.
    The English Physician Nicholas Culpeper; edited and with an introduction
by Michael A. Flannery.
        p.   cm.
    Originally published in 1708; reprinted, with minor revisions by the editor.
    Includes bibliographical references and index.
    ISBN-13: 978-0-8173-1558-0 (cloth: alk. paper)
    ISBN-10: 0-8173-1558-6 (alk. paper)
    1. Botany, Medical. 2. Materia medica—Early works to 1800. I. Flannery,
Michael A., 1953– II. Title.
    RS81C9   2007
    615'.321—dc22   2006024300

To Wayne Finley, PhD, MD,
for his love of and dedication to the history of medicine

CONTENTS

Preface

On the face of it, it seems odd that the first medical book published in the British North American colonies should be edited, introduced, and reprinted in the Deep South. It is, after all, really a piece of New England Americana. But this scarce little volume, the original a mere five and one-fourth inches high and ninety-four pages long, one of only five known copies, was part of the collection of Dr. Lawrence Reynolds, which today forms the core of the history of medicine library now bearing his name. The Reynolds Historical Library, officially dedicated on February 2, 1958, is located within the Lister Hill Library of the Health Sciences, University of Alabama at Birmingham.

That this diminutive compendium of remedies has not been reissued until now is somewhat surprising, especially given the fact that one of Culpeper's unmistakably genuine works and others that are attributed to him have been in constant publication since their author first penned them in the mid-seventeenth century. Yet, for reasons that will be explained in the introduction, this book has been overshadowed by the 1720 Boston reprinting of Culpeper's *Pharmacopoeia Londinensis or the London Dispensatory.* Much larger and more widely circulated, the *London Dispensatory* has clearly received much more attention. Nonetheless, the 1708 edition of *The English Physician* is a highly significant work—an interesting and in some ways unparalleled example of the transference of the Old World *materia medica* and medical theory to the New. The book provides a fascinating insight into the commercial dynamics emerging in the colonies as seen in the diligent efforts of its enterprising printer, Nicholas Boone, who was also responsible for publishing the more famous *London Dispensatory.* Paradoxically, the importation of this age-old materia medica via this Boston printing of *The English Physician* would set the stage for a new populist movement in health care that has appreciably affected

American medicine even to the present day. Distrustful of and disgusted with the arrogant presumptions and exorbitant fees of England's regular medical profession, Culpeper became at once a villain to physicians and a hero to the people. When similar medical rebels on this side of the Atlantic began looking for a historical champion, they turned to Culpeper.

Thus the present reprint is offered in the interest of revealing the strange and sometimes astonishing world of seventeenth- and eighteenth-century therapeutics and to make accessible the modest little volume that set forth a certain style and tone that became characteristic of American medical writing for generations to come. Perhaps the reprinting of this Alabama-owned copy of *The English Physician* is appropriate for another reason: It is a fact known by few that the state's very first medical school, the humble and short-lived Alabama Medical Institute of Wetumpka founded in 1844, itself was founded not by the "learned" regular medical profession but by botanic physicians as distrustful and disgusted with the medical elitists of their day as Culpeper had been with his. History always has its fitting ironies.

A Note on the Text

My GENERAL GOAL as editor of *The English Physician* has been to retain the original style and flavor of the work as much as possible. Thus, instances of "thee," "thy," and "thine" have not been replaced with their current pronoun equivalents. However, some modernization of spelling and punctuation has been employed to remove historical idiosyncrasies that would merely annoy the present-day reader. In that spirit, all instances of the so-called long s or medial s have been removed and replaced with a common s. In addition, some modernization of spelling has been employed, such as "oil" for the quainter "oyl," and so on.

The medical world of Culpeper and Boone was very different from our own, and extensive research was needed to make the pills, potions, plasters, decoctions, infusions, confections, electuaries, extracts, and myriad other dosage forms intelligible to the modern reader. It is hoped that the explanatory notes form a subtext and commentary to the work that render it accessible.

INTRODUCTION

O, mickle is the powerful grace that lies
In plants, herbs, stones, and their true qualities,
For naught so vile that on the earth doth live
But to the earth some special good doth give

SHAKESPEARE, *Romeo and Juliet*, ACT II, SCENE 3

For the earth which drinks in the rain that often comes upon it, and bears herbs
useful for those by whom it is cultivated, receives blessing from God.

HEBREWS 6:7 (NEW KING JAMES VERSION)

CONNECTIONS

SOME YEARS AGO there were two interesting PBS documentaries that covered in panoramic fashion the broad sweep of the history of science and technology: *Connections* (1978) and *The Day the Universe Changed* (1986). Although given to certain excesses intrinsic to the secular humanistic tendencies of their mercurial host, James Burke, the shows were, on the whole, marvelously clever and informative. In *Connections* Burke showed viewers how seemingly disparate advances in science and technology *were,* in fact, connected in some rather interesting ways. Indeed, these "connections" could be found in major discoveries of commonplace items now taken for granted. For example, he showed how a black viscous liquid oozing from distilled coal (coal tar) captured the interest of Friedrich Bayer and Friedrich Weskott. When they formed a dye-making company and employed the innovative Felix Hoffman as their chemist, he experimented with this waste product, ultimately yielding a stable compound called salicylic acid, from which today's common aspirin was synthesized.

Nicholas Culpeper, Nicholas Boone, and *The English Physician*, which Boone published in Boston in 1708, offer different but no less interesting "connections." How was it, for example, that ambitious entrepreneur Nicholas Boone decided to print the very first medical book in the British North American colonies? How was it that he selected not a learned treatise by one of the period's eminent physicians—Paré, Sydenham, or Harvey—but rather a modest little volume of medicinal recipes that he attributed to a rebel in clear opposition to the learned profession? How was it that the publication of this book would be prophetic in pointing toward a medical counterculture that flourishes in America to this very day? The answers to these questions shed light not only on the transference of medical knowledge from one side of the Atlantic to another but also on the life and contributions of Nicholas Culpeper—astrologer, herbalist, and practitioner of physic—who may readily be regarded as the morning star of alternative medicine in America. This points up yet another curious connection—with a "morning star" of a different kind, one of biblical proportions.

John Wycliffe and Nicholas Culpeper: Morning Stars of Reformations

John Wycliffe died in 1384, 232 years before Culpeper was born.[1] Nevertheless, the two were kindred spirits. An independent thinker, Wycliffe capitalized on the papal schism of 1378 to challenge religious orthodoxy by proclaiming Rome corrupt and its doctrines wicked. The learned CARDINAL elite he dubbed with the derisive acronym "Captain of the Apostates of the Realm of the Devil, Impudent and Nefarious Ally of Lucifer."[2] Not so much a systematic religious thinker as an expositor of institutional corruption, social abuse, and biblical error, Wycliffe challenged the church's claim to absolute authority and mocked such priestly pretensions as absurd and unscriptural. The Bible should be the church's sole authority, he argued, and his insistence that the Bible should be translated into the language of the people instead of kept in the Latin Vulgate of the ruling class fit in well with ideas such as the doctrine of a priesthood of all believers that became the cornerstone of the Reformation two hundred years later.

Wycliffe soon built a following called Lollards (originally a derisive term meaning "mumblers"), who disseminated his ideas and eventually managed to carry out their leader's wish in translating the entire Bible from Latin into English. An earlier, more literal translation eventually gave way to a posthumous version in 1388 that modern editor W. R. Cooper has called "a superior, powerful rendition of the Scriptures."[3] Despite persecution, the persistence of the Lollards bore fruit in numerous texts of what soon became known as *The Wycliffe Bible*.[4] From these texts came glossed Gospels, sermon cycles, and doctrinal tracts that would change the face of Christendom forever. When Bohemian King Wencelas IV's sister, Anne, married Richard II of England in 1382, ideas from the British Isles began filtering into the Continent, and John Huss soon found himself captivated by the ideas of Wycliffe. Huss would pay with his life for those ideas, but his reformist views à la Wycliffe influenced a German cleric-turned-iconoclast named Martin Luther. No wonder, then, that Wycliffe has been widely regarded as "the morning star of the Reformation."

Nicholas Culpeper was a similar figure. Born on October 18, 1616, to a recently widowed mother, the boy grew up with his own ideas, ideas that seemingly no institution (whether Cambridge, where he failed his medical studies, or the Apothecary Society in London, by which he was not licensed) could tame. By nature he was rebellious and eagerly questioned convention. In religion he favored the nonconformists and fought in the British Civil War for Oliver Cromwell's Parliamentarians against King Charles I's Cavaliers; in medicine he challenged the establishment by doing the unthinkable—translating the 1618 *Pharmacopoeia Londinensis* from Latin into English, which he published as the *Physical Directory* in 1649. By 1652 he had published a folio,

The English Physitian: or an Astrological Discourse on the Vulgar Herbs of this Nation, which is now popularly known as Culpeper's *Herbal* and remains in print to this day. In 1653, to the disgust of the Royal College of Physicians, he published a translation of the second edition of the *Pharmacopoeia Londinensis.*[5] Four months and five days later, on January 10, 1654, he died of consumption (pulmonary tuberculosis) at his home in Spitalfields, just a few miles northeast of London. He was only thirty-eight years old, but during his brief lifetime he had caused quite a stir among the elitist physicians of his day.

In order to appreciate the revolutionary character of Culpeper's work, one must realize that until very recently medicine was more art than science. Members of the medical establishment of Culpeper's generation may indeed have felt their therapeutics were efficacious and the best available given the current state of knowledge; indeed, their often-expressed belief that there was an abundant supply of quacks and charlatans all too willing to pick an ailing public's pocket contained more than a hint of truth. But the "best available" treatment was often not much in seventeenth- and eighteenth-century England. To counterbalance this embarrassingly obvious limitation, physicians often based their claims to authority on little more than lofty credentials, complex and sometimes convoluted theories, and elaborate nosologies. Furthermore, the medical profession's pecuniary interests were often privileged over their patients' well-being. Members of London's aristocratic College of Physicians wanted a monopoly on health care and consequently sought to keep their complicated and obtuse therapies hidden from the people; the best way to do that was to write their texts and compendia in Latin. Moreover, they sought to ensure their commercial interests with a law that required all practitioners within a seven-mile radius of the city to be licensed with the college. Culpeper knew what they were up to and would have none of it.[6]

The apothecaries were not much better, selling drugs at an average profit of 300 percent.[7] The physicians' and apothecaries' rather flagrant impositions upon the people's meager incomes were especially irksome to Culpeper, since he could see plants growing under his feet, free for the taking, that he was convinced had medicinal virtues equal and sometimes superior to the rare exotics promoted by the medical profession. Culpeper blasted the college for cloaking its "cures" in the secret language of the learned, and in his second edition of the *Physical Directory* charged: "All your skill in physick might have been written in the inside of a ring. . . . Colledg, colledg, thou art diseased, the cause is mammon. The diagnostics are these: *Ipse dixit,* seven miles about London, lay him in prison: Be as proud as Lucifer, ride in state with a foot-cloth, love the sight of angels [coins], cheat the rich, neglect the poor, do nothing without money, be self-conceited, be angry."[8]

Culpeper added injury to insult by strongly criticizing some of the medicines of the *Pharmacopoeia*. In his translation of the *Pharmacopoeia Londinensis* (first edition) he bemoaned the instructions for making *Mel Helleboratum* (hellebore with honey) and gave an assessment that would survive for centuries: "What a *monstrum horrendum,* horrible, terrible recipe have we got here:—A pound of white hellebore boiled in fourteen pounds of water to seven. . . . Imagine the hellebore still remaining in its vigour after being so long tired out with a tedious boiling (for less boiling would boil an ox), what should the medicine do? Purge melancholy, say they. But from whom? From men or beasts? The devil would not take it unless it were poured down his throat with a horn."[9] He lost none of his biting wit and sarcasm in his translation of the second edition. Of Water and Spirit of Earthworms, he complained, "Tis a mess altogether, it may be they [the members of the college] intended it for a universal medicine."[10] Ointment of Elencampane with Quicksilver (that is, mercury) drew this clever if not telling response: "My opinion of this ointment, is (briefly) this: It was invented for the itch, without quick-silver it will do no good, with quick-silver it may do harm."[11] Culpeper was quick to point out when the college recommended a remedy largely for its high price. For example, of *Aqua Gilbertii* (Gilbert's Water), he said derisively, "I suppose this was invented for a cordial to strengthen the heart, to relieve languishing nature. It is exceeding dear. I forbear the dose, they that have money enough to make it themselves, cannot want time to study both the virtues and dose. I would have gentlemen to be studious."[12]

Defenders of the *Pharmacopoeia,* mostly members of the College of Physicians and their rich patrons, lost no time in sending back volleys of vituperation. Not amused by the impudence of this persona non grata, the royalist paper *Mercurius Pragmaticus* charged, "The Pharmacopoeia was done very filthily into English by one Nicholas Culpeper . . . and by two years drunken labour hath gallimaufried the apothecaries book into nonsense, mixing every receipt therein with some scruples, at least, of rebellion or atheism, besides the danger of poisoning men's bodies."[13] Nonetheless, the college was careful not to give too much attention to this Spitalfields upstart. "Officially," observes Culpeper's most recent biographer, "the College's response was dignified silence. Unofficially, dissecting knives were drawn."[14] College physicians accused Culpeper of being a fraud and an empiric, the latter term implying he had no grasp of theory and no grounding in the "higher" and more "learned" tenets of the healing art. Sarcastic rhymes were composed attacking the presumptuous astrologer-healer from Spitalfields:

This man indee's the *Vicar* of St. *Fools*
Yet contradicts *Physitians* and the *Schoolls*
And with a handful of conceited knowledge . . .
Dare challenge all the Doctors in the Colledge."[15]

William Johnson, chemist for the college, called Culpeper to the challenge: "And for your judgment in physic, I know you dare not come thither to the test."[16]

The accusations were enough to cast Culpeper far and firm from the pale of medical orthodoxy. For years thereafter he was regarded as a scoundrel and a quack. In an address to the Massachusetts Medical Society in 1869, the venerable physician Oliver Wendell Holmes indicted Culpeper as "a shrewd charlatan, and as impudent a varlet as ever prescribed for a colic; but knew very well what he was about, and badgers the College with great vigor."[17] More than fifty years later historians continued to vilify the English herbalist as an ignorant "quacksalver."[18]

It is significant to point out that opinion of the learned college notwith standing, practitioners in the American colonies tended to see Culpeper in a different light. Copies of many Culpeper works, but mostly his *English Physician,* came across the Atlantic to adorn the bookshelves of both wealthy and modest households. "It was Culpeper," affirms one modern authority, "who reached furthest into the everyday lives of Englishmen in the New World."[19] More important, his books could be found in many a New England physician-preacher's library. In today's age of rigorous medical school entrance exams and strict licensure, it is easy to forget that health care provision was much more fluid throughout most of history. Beyond the seven-mile radius of London, for example, formally trained physicians were scarce, and apothecaries had been accorded full practicing rights equal with physicians since 1703.[20] In the British American colonies, where there was a serious lack of formally trained physicians, most health care was provided in the home or in towns and cities by apothecaries or ministers. The clergy, in fact, provided an important stopgap in an otherwise underpopulated field of professional care. It has been noted that popular images of dour clerics hunched over Bible texts and commentaries by candlelight preparing endless sermons castigating the flock for their sinfulness are less accurate than more wholesome scenes of God's servants consoling the sick and tending to their needs.[21] The absence of physicians in the colonies, the biblical injunctions to visit and heal the sick, and the need for most clergy to supplement their modest stipends helped establish the preacher-physician as a viable and sometimes prominent part of community health care. It is interesting to note that in an analysis of nineteen New England divines who also had medical interests, Nicholas Culpeper's works predominated in their personal libraries.[22] "It is hardly surprising," writes historian Patricia Watson, "that Culpeper's writings (as well as those of [William] Salmon), so firmly entrenched in the antiroyalist, anti-monopolistic polemic of his day, were so popular among Puritan ministers of New England."[23] Indeed, there are indications that Culpeper health guides were popular outside the region as well; inventories suggest that his books were commonplace on the library shelves of Virginia's gentry.[24]

But the herbalist from Spitalfields had an influence that extended beyond the colonial period. The reasons are found in the nature of early American health care itself. The status of physicians was never especially high in the New World. The purging, puking, and bleeding of patients often seemed to know no bounds, a disquieting fact that relegated calling in the doctor to the means of last resort. Besides, it was expensive and often not very efficacious. War and America's victory over the crown seemed to cast the effete English physicians and their arrogant posturings in an even worse light, and some began to wonder if their pompous colleagues in Philadelphia, Boston, and elsewhere in the young Republic were any better. Was it really necessary to license and recognize such pretense in a nation whose newfound freedoms should also include the freedom of therapeutic choice? Samuel Thomson answered with a resounding no. His *New Guide to Health, or, Botanic Family Physician,* first published in 1822, echoed Culpeper's theme of "every man his own physician."

Others soon followed to create a persistent voice of opposition to the regular medical establishment. Wooster Beach, a New York physician disgruntled with his colleagues' approach to medicine, came under the influence of an herbalist named Jacob Tidd. So convinced was Beach of the wisdom of nature's remedies that he left the orthodox flock to found his Reformed Medical Academy in 1829. This would evolve into the American Eclectics, a botanical group that challenged regular medicine into the twentieth century. Another proponent of botanical medicine was Alva Curtis, Thomson's erstwhile protégé, who established the Physio-Medicals in 1838.[25] Like Culpeper, these groups shunned the expensive and sometimes harmful medicines of the regulars in favor of botanical remedies and became in their own right the people's doctors. Like Culpeper, they too opposed mainstream medicine's attempts to create a monopoly through restrictive licensing and other regulatory measures.

The American botanics knew and appreciated their role as Culpeper's progeny. Elias Smith, a Bostonian who had a rather shaky relationship with Samuel Thomson but remained a persistent and vocal spokesman for the botanic cause, relied heavily upon Culpeper and kept an original edition of

The English Physician in his personal library.[26] Eclectic physician Alexander Wilder gave a detailed, if somewhat factually inaccurate, account of Culpeper's contributions to the healing art in his partisan history of medicine, concluding that the English champion of herbalism was "a liberal scholar as well as a broad thinker."[27] John Uri Lloyd, perhaps the most famous Eclectic and most notable American pharmacognosist of the late nineteenth and early twentieth centuries, used "many editions" of Culpeper in compiling his history of U.S. pharmacopoeial drugs.[28] Like so many Protestants who followed in the footsteps of Wycliffe—indeed, who followed *because* of Wycliffe's Bible—medical "Protestants" in America followed Culpeper's lead in eschewing the pretensions of baseless authority, secrecy, and monopoly in favor of more accessible and affordable health care based upon remedies they genuinely believed to be better for the people.[29] "Thus God *has, in his infinite goodness,*" declared Wooster Beach in his Eclectic manifesto, "*brought into existence a more rational system of medicine, in the place of one productive of pernicious consequences; a system which heals disease with remedies more in conformity with the intentions of nature, and re-establishes health without destroying the source of life.* The reader," he added, "will at once perceive the propriety of a work calculated to effect a change, or introduce a reformation, in the noble science of medicine."[30] Culpeper could have easily written these lines. It is important to note that these medical "Protestants" were no more shunning science than Wycliffe was shunning doctrine. But if Wycliffe is the analogous figure to Culpeper, then who played Lollard for the medical rebel from Spitalfields? Who spread his brand of medical populism to American shores? Answer: his printers.

CULPEPER COMES TO AMERICA

There is little question that Culpeper became many a printer's cash cow. Peter Cole, John Streater, Nathaniel Brooke, and Obadiah Blagrave all sold first or early editions of Culpeper's works at considerable profit. His *English Physician* filled a much-needed gap in health care for the poor—at only 3 pence per copy, written in plain English, with many simple and easily prepared remedies, this self-help guide was indispensable to people of more modest means, who were eager to include it among their few possessions.[31] In fact, the book sold so well that one historian has suggested that "Culpeper worked mainly for London booksellers, who paid him for the full rights of his work on completion, and . . . the booksellers both set and satisfied the market for his editions."[32] This assessment seems a bit overdrawn, however. Culpeper clearly relished his work, fervently believed in what he wrote, and was good at what he did; the mere fact that his works sold well should not imply that he was the printers' lackey or slave any more than *any* popular author is beholden to the publisher who provides a ready and handsome income. It seems more likely that the relationship was symbiotic rather than servile.

In any case, popularity and controversy combined to considerably complicate the Culpeper bibliography. The Culpeper name was so well known and so valuable, in fact, that bootlegged editions of his books appeared even in his own lifetime, and the author took great pains to alert his readers to the counterfeits. Not surprisingly, a flurry of assorted posthumous publications under the Culpeper—and sometimes "Culpepper"—banner soon followed. Even his widow and her new husband, a "mystical cheat"[33] by the name of John Heydon, tried to cash in on the Culpeper name with numerous spurious "additions" to the Culpeper bibliography. Alice Culpeper claimed that her deceased husband left behind some "79 books" in manuscript form.[34] Although we have only her word for this, her husband's untimely death did not stop her from trying to keep the cachet of the Culpeper name alive. Before grass could sprout on her husband's grave in the New Bethlehem churchyard, she and husband-to-be Heyden attempted to sell a nostrum called Aurum Potable under Culpeper's endorsement. Then in May of 1655, Nathaniel Brooke rushed *Culpeper's Last Legacy* to press. The publication came prefaced with an alleged letter of authenticity from his widow, which brought forth her furious denial.[35] It seems likely that the ambitious Mrs. Culpeper may have disavowed her *Last Legacy* missive for Brooke because she had struck a deal with Peter Cole to promote her "drinkable gold" potion. At any rate she released a work printed by Cole shortly thereafter titled *Mr. Culpeper's Treatise of Aurum*

Potable, which included an attack upon Brooke. Alice's protests notwithstanding, Brooke was undaunted. Two years later he was still issuing the *Last Legacy*
with the letter unamended. A. Culpeper (aka Nathaniel Brooke?) insisted to
the Culpeper faithful that the book's contents were genuine:

> Having in my Hands these my Husbands last experiences in Physick
> and Chyurgery, & c. composed out of his daily practice, which he laid a
> severe injunction on me to publish for the generall good after his
> decease; therefore to stop the mouths of malicious Persons, who may be
> apt to abuse and slander his labours, and to discharge that duty and
> debt of gratitude due to his name from one so neerly related to him, I
> do hereby testifie that the Copy of what is here printed is truly and real-
> ly his own, and was delivered to my trust among his choicest secrets
> upon his death-bed, and I do further approve the printing thereof, and
> having viewed them see nothing in them but what is his own. To the
> truth of all which I do here subscribe my hand.
>
> A. Culpeper[36]

Whether authorized by Alice or not, the work almost certainly is not a
Nicholas Culpeper production. There is a counterfeit quality to this book. It
consists of a hodgepodge of treatises and expositions on various subjects and
ailments, with proposed remedies ranging from simples (that is, single plants
of single medicinal action prepared simply) to remedies for simpletons, as
when it is suggested that "shaking palsey" can be cured by smelling one's
toes.[37] It went from silly to sillier when Nicholas's erstwhile printer Peter Cole
claimed to be in possession of a letter by none other than Culpeper's ghost!
He published it in 1656 as "Mr. Culpeper's Ghost, giving seasonable advice to
lovers of his writings."[38] Indeed, one recent biographer has noted, "He was
even more prolific dead than alive."[39]

It should come as little surprise, then, that Culpeper soon caught the eye of
an enterprising printer in the American colonies. In 1708 Nicholas Boone
issued from his print shop "at the corner of School-House-Lane" the book that

would be widely regarded by historians and medical bibliographers as the first medical book published in the British American colonies: *The English Physician. Containing, Admirable and Approved Remedies, for Several of the Most Usual Diseases.*[40] The book is *not* a genuine Culpeper production but rather a reprinting (word for word, in fact) of the *Physical Receipts, or, The New English Physician* first published by Thomas Howkins in London in 1690.[41] More will be said about this in the next section, but the question begs to be asked: why this and not the more popular and genuine *English Physician* or even *English Physician Enlarged?* The simplest answer is probably the most plausible: this is what Boone had on hand. In an age before real copyright, reprintings and clever reassemblings of works under attributed authors were commonplace. The only protection against piracy of titles was accorded to printers—*not* authors—through a weak and often ignored Stationers' Register.

Thus, Nicholas Boone would not have been averse to publishing a book under the name of an author readily known to the citizens of Boston. After all, he had competition; by the early 1700s Boston had become busy with printers and booksellers. From 1645 to 1711 there were no fewer than thirty bookshops in the vicinity of Boston's Town House or Exchange, Boone's among them.[42] But why publish a book of medicinal recipes? There is evidence that Boone had at least some association with apothecaries early on. On April 24, 1704, not quite twenty-five years of age, he issued the city's first newspaper, *The Boston News-Letter,* at his print shop next to Major Davis's Apothecary.[43] Certainly common pleasantries must have been exchanged and some general business banter passed between the young printer and his neighbor. Books, booksellers, printers, and the apothecary's art seemed to mix often, if not always well. In the 1670s, Joseph Tappin conducted a book business and added "an apothecary's department," said to be the first in New England.[44] One of Boone's competitors, Samuel Sewell, had at one time unsuccessfully apprenticed to an apothecary, Samuel Checkley.[45] Boone knew Checkley and worked closely with him on city affairs.[46] Apothecaries in Boston were apt to be looking for a handy guide to medicines, and if it came in more accessible English (their Latin might well have been a bit shaky), so much the better. Add to this a sizeable clientele from clergy (who, as we already saw, prized Culpeper as a medical guide), and the choice of a "Culpeper" volume of some kind makes sense.

Publishing this ninety-four-page book was a printer's dream. Brief, requiring no illustrations or special marks, its reissue promised minimal investment of time and resources. But Howkins's *Physical Receipts* was less well known than the famous herbal. So a simple adjustment in title, carrying forward Howkins's attribution of "N. Culpepper" (the double p spelling was a common mistake of printers), seems like a perfectly understandable business decision for the enterprising Mr. Boone. If his willingness to play fast and loose with the herbalist's name and work seems distasteful to our modern sensibilities, it must be remembered that the practice was common and no stranger to health guides of the period.[47] The sheer number and variety of posthumous Culpeper titles—real or attributed—can only be described as a veritable frenzy of printing press activity.

Interestingly, the only known copy of *Physical Receipts* in the British Library (formerly British Museum) is incomplete. Arranged alphabetically, its abrupt ending on page 64 at the "King's Evil" suggests a considerable portion missing. A careful comparison with Boone's *English Physician* indicates it is a verbatim reissue of the work; although the latter goes on to include "Liver and Lungs Infirmities." The *English Physician* is, in fact, only a few pages longer (three to be exact) than its earlier twin. We know from the addition of "Finis" on page 94 of the original that the volume is complete or at least as complete as Boone intended it to be. Both books' scarcity (there are only five extant cataloged copies of the Boston *English Physician* of 1708)[48] may be attributed to the ready-reference nature of both. These were designed to be used and used often. Their likely proximity to boiling pots, simmering medicinal stews, draining colanders, and similar apparatus must have exacted its toll. The loss of Boone's shop in a fire in 1711 might have destroyed any remaining stock supply in his shop.[49]

Ever resilient, Nicholas rebuilt his business. We might infer the success of his first effort at publishing a medical book by the fact that he published the colony's second one in 1720, this time a genuine Culpeper title—the *London Dispensatory*—a much more extensive work and a more ambitious printer's project. His contributions to medical firsts did not end there; he apparently decided also to follow in Joseph Tappin's footsteps and engage in selling medicine in his bookshop (interestingly, just when he was simultaneously selling his *English Physician*), for on October 4, 1708, he printed the first patent medicine advertisement in America by announcing for sale at his shop "at the Sign of the Bible near the corner of School-House-Lane" the famed remedy "Daffy's Elixir Salutis, very good, at four shillings and six-pence per half pint Bottle."[50] Predictably, "Doctor Anthony Daffey's [sic] Original Elixir Salutis" appeared again in the *Boston News-Letter*, coinciding nicely with the appearance of Boone's *London Dispensatory*.[51] With his business acumen, Boone rose to prominence in Boston's public and social life. Upon his death in November of 1738 he left an estate valued at 1,981 pounds, the modern-day equivalent of slightly over 355,000 dollars.[52]

THE ENGLISH PHYSICIAN IN CONTEXT

Of course, none of the preceding discussion really addresses the need for reprinting a little book under one hundred pages issued primarily to satisfy the financial interests of an ambitious Boston printer and bookseller. If rarity and value are points favoring a reprint, this book certainly meets the test. When historian David Cowen first alerted the public to it in 1956, he thought the Boston Medical Library owned the only complete copy.[53] Since then more have surfaced, but only a handful. The value of such a volume is hard to estimate. In 2001 Nicholas Boone's much more prevalent 1720 *London Dispensatory* sold for 22,000 dollars.[54] Adjustments for rarity and primacy would suggest a much higher value for *The English Physician*. But value and scarcity can hardly serve as the sole justification for offering an old book to a new public. There must be more.

Historians have generally been dismissive of *The English Physician*. Mary Rhinelander McCarl, commenting upon the popular practice of attributing health guides posthumously to Culpeper, referred to Howkins's *Physical*

Receipts, from which Boone's printing was drawn, as one among many "undifferentiated collections of herbal cures at the low end of the market."[55] Suggesting that *The English Physician* barely warranted the title of a "book," Cowen characterized the Boston work as largely composed of domestic remedies and "obviously intended for the layman."[56] He went on to pay much more attention to Boone's 1720 publication, calling it "far more important [than the 1708 *English Physician*]. . . . This is a very significant book: not only was it the first full-length medical work published in the colonies," he added, "but it was also the first work of a pharmacopoeial or dispensatory nature."[57] Cowen's assessment of the *London Dispensatory* is superficially correct—it *was* a far more substantial work—but a careful perusal of the earlier title suggests something much more than a mere domestic health guide for the commoner.

A comparative examination of *The English Physician* with Culpeper's other works reveals not just another permutation of his herbal (though there are a significant number of botanical remedies, as there were in *all* compendia at that time) but rather a condensed, combined, and "modified" version of the *Physical Directory* and his *London Dispensatory,* with some simples from the *English Physitian* thrown in. Examples of some fairly complex polypharmacy concoctions are easy to find: *Electuarium Reginæ Coloniens,* for example, is a complex concoction of highly exotic products, the recipe for curing the French pox (syphilis) would challenge the most well-stocked and accomplished apothecary, and Ungent sumac is much more than sumac leaves put into a simple ointment. These were largely remedies approved by Culpeper taken from the official *Pharmacopoeia Londinensis,* but a careful examination of the text will expose several places where the given remedy does not even appear in a Culpeper work. That said, it would be too harsh to say the volume bears no relationship to Culpeper, because in other places the recipes are clearly paraphrases or complete borrowings of known Culpeper writings. The best that can be offered is that *The English Physician* issued by Boone was in the style of its attributed author. It *was,* after all, in English; contained something of the flavor of Culpeper's commentary, sans the vituperation against the college; and at least claimed to be "fitted to the meanest capacity."

But those purchasing it for home use were likely to be disappointed when they found that to heal an "inward bruise" they needed some resin from the fruits of East Indian climbing palms and ground-up mummy—yes, mummy! Likewise, they were probably left rather nonplussed when they discovered that joint ache and numbness needed a drachm of Mithridate, a polypharmacy concoction that included opium and some *fifty different ingredients*. Rather than becoming hypnotized by the name Culpeper into thinking the work is just a variation on his familiar theme of domestic healing, it is much more accurate to see the book for what it really is: a blending of herbal remedies with a kind of synopsis in the style of Culpeper's *Physical Directory*, which might hint at the reason for Howkins's selection of *Physical Receipts* for the title of the original work.

But if it was not really intended for those "of the meanest capacity," whom *did* Boone intend it for? Probably the book would have quickly caught the eye of apothecaries, clergy, and others with the ways and means to acquire such expensive and sometimes exotic articles. Those not instructed by God or the profession in the arcane art of healing would have found their household gardens wholly inadequate to the task; trips to the apothecary shop were unquestionably necessary to get many of the articles required in this book. From Boone's standpoint, as a man rising in the community and with social aspirations to connect with those of a more "proper" station, his *English Physician* would have been just the ticket. If an interested housewife of more middling means wanted the book for some of the simples it contained, so much the better. After all, *none* of them had seen a production quite like it in the colonies unless it was an expensive import, so he had a ready market. These motives seem very unlike Culpeper and rather unbefitting his name. But on the other hand he was being brought among friends. Wealthy or poor, virtually everyone in Boston in the early eighteenth century was Culpeper's religious brethren, staunch Puritans and "nonconformists" to the last man, woman, and child. Thus, that it carried the name Culpeper established the book as a "Puritan-friendly" publication. By 1708 Culpeper had become a name synonymous with open inquiry and self-help, distrustful of princely authority and a standard-bearer for empirical application (efficacy would certainly go too far) rather than the slavish adherence to the secret theories of rank and privilege.

The deceptively simple but nonetheless complex character of the 1708 *English Physician* speaks to its importance. More than just a common herbalist's guide, this book is truly reflective of the therapeutics of the day. In order to understand the implications of this, it is necessary to review seventeenth- and eighteenth-century ideas about disease. For centuries disease theory was dominated by Galen, a renowned second-century physician who served as personal physician to Emperor Marcus Aurelius. Extrapolating from an earlier Greek healer, Empedocles, who saw the universe as composed of four elements—earth, air, fire, and water—Galen viewed disease as the product of an imbalance of "humors," which were composed of blood, phlegm, black bile, and yellow bile. Thus, the key to eliminating disease resided in the healer's ability to "adjust" these humors through bleeding, sweating, purging, or puking the patient back to health. This could be done through venesection (opening a vein for bloodletting) or scarification (making small superficial incisions to release smaller amounts of blood and "putrefaction"). It could also be done with the administration of assorted medicines principally made from a variety of plants, though occasionally animal and mineral products were used. These would "rebalance" other humors in various and sometimes rather unpleasant ways like sweating, purging, or puking. The correlation between a plant and its properties was its taste; plants could be sweet, dry, acid, or neutral, with each affecting a particular humor in a particular way. Generations of physicians spent whole careers outlining and detailing these alleged properties by postulating, proposing, and sometimes arguing about what plant was good for what humor and what illness derived from what "bad" humor. Thus, when the physician's bloodletting tools were not out, rest assured that some botanical was being strained, siphoned, macerated, mixed, brewed, or boiled to correct the malady.

In the first half of the sixteenth century another authority came along to challenge the preeminence of Galenic theory. He was a Swiss-born physician named Theophrastus Bombastus von Hohenheim, better known as Paracelsus. He extrapolated from the ancient and arcane art of alchemy to introduce various chemicals into the armamentarium against disease. For Paracelsus disease was the product of so-called acrimonies (an imbalance of alkaline or acid) that affected the *archeus,* or life force. Half scientist, half mystic, Paracelsus provided the foundation that his followers (especially François de le Boë Sylvius) developed into a theory of iatrochemical principles that involved bringing the archeus back into balance with mineral rather than botanical agents.[58] Whether Galenic or Paracelsian theories were practiced, in the end it mattered little; disease was in either case a systemic problem, a matter of correcting a maladjusted internal property within the body.

By Culpeper's day these therapeutic currents had coalesced into a mixture of "Galenics" (essentially botanically based remedies) and minerals harkening to the Paracelsian school of thought. Medicine was also infused with mysticism, which included astrology. Culpeper knew the most important astrologist of his day, William Lilly, and believed that plants were ruled by certain planets and that their therapeutic qualities were affected by the time of harvesting, preparing, and administering them. Although he was derided for his astrological inclinations by the college and by later historians,[59] Culpeper was not alone in thinking that the heavens influenced health and healing in appreciable ways. The learned William Harvey, whose *De motu cordis* (1628) gave us the first accurate description of the heart and circulatory system, subscribed to astrology, as did most every patient.[60] Though waning, the credibility of astrology carried into the next century, and that one believed in it by no means presented a bar to scientific advancement. The eminent French astronomer Joseph-Nicolas Delisle, for example, earned a pension making astrological prognostications for the regency prior to his appointment as chair of mathematics at the Collège Royal in 1718.[61] Nonetheless, Culpeper's discussion of remedies is largely unaffected by his astrological inclinations, and the two can easily be separated without essential loss. This is clearly evident in the book in hand, as it contains little hint of celestial influence even though it retains all of the stylistic trappings of its attributed author.

More down to earth, the evidence we have of early eighteenth-century therapeutics fits neatly within the context of *The English Physician*. It is interesting to note that a survey of four typical New England practitioners from the mid- to late 1700s reveals that their top five medicinal agents of choice were all imported and, with the exception of cantharides (a beetle), all botanical.[62] Besides imported remedies these physicians prescribed more common items familiar to every British citizen, such as honey, lavender, chamomile, marshmallow, larch oil, rhubarb, elderberry, barley, tormentil, and ivy. Each of these can also be found in *The English Physician*. Of course, this survey data of physicians and their therapeutic behaviors postdates Boone's publication by some fifty years, but the more things change the more they stay the same. By mid-century Galenism was slowly yielding to more "sophisticated" theories, but the basic treatments and materia medica remained unaltered. "Although strict humoralism was being replaced . . . by concepts of excessive or diminished nervous or vascular tension ('solidism')," explains J. Worth Estes, "the therapeutic principles of their treatment, by restoring balance or tension, were similar."[63] Therefore, it is fair to conclude that the regimens found in Boone's little compendium are reflective of the general therapeutics then prevailing in England and its North American colonies.

It is worth repeating that this book is also important because it introduced to America a brand of health care that spoke to the masses (in form if not always in content), one that was distinctly populist and wary of the hubris of orthodox medicine. As we have seen, Culpeper was in some ways the precursor of an American botanical movement that served as a persistent counter to regular medicine and thus in some measure forced scientific and professional advances in the medical establishment. Without the obstreperous voice of these American botanics to challenge and pressure the regular physicians, it is quite likely that much progress would have been stultified by complacency. Indeed, that voice grew increasingly loud in the nineteenth century until it reached a climax in the American Civil War.[64] It may be asserted with some confidence that it started here; it started with Nicholas Boone's Boston printing of *The English Physician*.

To some extent this medical populism is still with us today in the trend toward botanical alternatives to modern pharmaceuticals. The current interest has even received legislative sanction in the immensely popular Dietary Supplement Health and Education Act (DSHEA) passed in 1994, a law enacted to protect herbals and similar products from the costly regulatory demands required of standard prescription and over-the-counter drugs. The DSHEA reflected far more than just an aberration or fad. Its sponsor, Senator Orrin Hatch, observed that his opponents were powerful (paralleling the College of Physicians in Culpeper's day), most notably in the government's Food and Drug Administration.[65] But, like Culpeper, he also had powerful allies: the "more than 100 million Americans who regularly use dietary supplements [herbs]. . . . Members received more letters, calls and visits about our bill . . . than about any other issue before Congress."[66] The DSHEA stands today as a testimony to Culpeper's therapeutic populism.

Culpeper's most recent biographer put it nicely:

> What Culpeper did was challenge the principle that medical knowledge belonged solely to physicians—indeed that expert knowledge of any sort belonged to the experts. He helped to reveal a division that has yet to heal, between orthodox and alternative medicine, between professional expertise and personal empowerment. He would probably have deplored many of the practices that currently take place in the name of "alternative medicine"—he would have considered Chinese or Indian remedies, for example, as being out of place in the northern European or North American clime. But he would recognize the current controversies over medicine as the same ones he was engaged in 350 years ago."[67]

One final aspect to this book needs to be emphasized: While the book includes complicated remedies, as mentioned before, it *also* contains its share of simples. These simples speak as much to the significance of this book as do the more complex preparations. In spite of Alexander Wilder's consistent inability to get his facts straight concerning his hero, which includes his according Culpeper vaunted status as author of the first English herbal (a distinction more accurately belonging to the *Leech Book of Bald* [AD 900–950])[68] as well as his consistent misspelling of Culpepper, he *did* point up the genuinely unique botanical transformation that Culpeper wrought upon the American scene. As nature's English apothecary was planted in and around Boston, whether in homely gardens, rectory plots, wealthy courtyards, or druggists' nurseries, some plants inevitably escaped their cultivated moorings to scatter across the land—and scatter they *did*—effecting a remarkable and permanent metamorphosis of the American landscape. In short, these plants spread in profusion. "We find many of them at the present time [1904] equally common in America," declared Wilder, "and frequently used as medicines. Among them are, agrimony, avens, bittersweet, nightshade, gentian, flowerde-luce, cleavers, comfrey, pennyroyal, dandelion, mullein, poplar bark, willow, catmint, thoroughwort, eyebright. Quaint and antique as the work [*The English Physician*] may be, it contains much information of great utility."[69] Wilder's claim is substantiated by the large number of introduced, naturalized, and adventive plants found in *The English Physician* (see the appendix).

Taken altogether, the modest appearance of the small, plain, unillustrated *English Physician* belies its significance in the history of American medical bibliography. The book deserves long overdue recognition for at least four important reasons: (1) It was the first medical book published in the British North American colonies; (2) Its brief but varied contents reflect the general therapeutics of colonial America both domestic *and* professional; (3) It presaged a long and enduring alternative medicine movement in America that is in some measure still alive today; and (4) It undoubtedly served as a catalyst for significant botanical introductions of Old World flora into the New World, permanently transforming the American landscape.

CONCLUSION

Perhaps it is best to conclude this introduction with the connections theme that opened it. If we can see connections between Wycliffe and his Lollards and Culpeper and his printers, and between Wycliffe's religious Protestantism and Culpeper's medical protestantism, perhaps other connections can be found as well. Ironically, disease becomes another connective link. The so-called Black Death of 1346–61 weakened the church materially and spiritually. Materially, the Black Death wiped out nearly a whole generation of clergy and spiritually, it made the church appear impotent in the face of what looked like providential judgment for its worldly lapses. Riding the crest of this plague-ridden wave, Wycliffe and his Lollards were the first to navigate Europe toward Protestantism. Martin Luther's Reformation, which, as we have seen, was sparked by the influence of Huss, who was, in turn, influenced by Wycliffe, bore a direct link with the English Puritanism that had so influenced the nonconformist Culpeper and his brethren who chose to sail to the New World. "Thus it is not too much to claim," write historians Frederick Cartwright and Michael Biddiss, "that the Protestant Reformation, the sailing of the Brownist Pilgrim Fathers in the *Mayflower* on 6 September 1620 . . . can all be linked with the deviation from established religion that followed the disaster of the Black Death."[70]

The Great Plague of London of 1665, just a few years after Culpeper's death, did for medicine what the Black Death did for religion. Utterly defenseless against the *Yersinia pestis* (formerly *Pasteurella pestis*) bacteria, which they did not understand or even recognize, physicians lost caste with their patients, furthering the populist impulse in medicine. At least Daniel Defoe thought so. He wrote of the Great Plague, "[L]et all the Prescriptions of all the Physicians in *London* be examined; and it will be found, with such Variations only, as the particular Fancy of the Doctor leads him to; so that . . . every Man judging a little of his own Constitution and manner of his living, and Circumstances of his being infected, may direct his own medicines out of the ordinary Drugs and Preparations."[71] This attitude exemplifies the book reprinted here. Whether one harvested from the homely garden in one's back-yard or bought from the more expensive and complicated preparations of the apothecary, it was *The English Physician* that served as its owner's vade mecum, an ever-present guide to care and therapeutic choice unmediated by a professional.

In the final analysis, the story of the first medical book ever published in

British North America is the story of European and American history itself: of plagues and protestants (clerical and clinical), of Bibles and booksellers, of "learned" physicians and medical "philistines," of dogmatists and their dogmas versus reformists and their reforms. It is equally a message of concern for and interest in the people's welfare. Culpeper's concern for the masses was genuine, and his struggles to promote health and healing for his fellow citizens high and low were dogged and determined. In his preface—we can forget for the moment that although it was not penned by Culpeper it *was* certainly in his style—he touchingly exhorts his reader: "Be kind and good to your Poor Neighbour, for which you may expect the Blessing of God." Wycliffe, whose advocacy for his compatriots' souls was as zealous as the English herbalist's pleading for their bodies, echoes Culpeper in his Bible: "And, brethren, we pray you, reprove ye unpeaceable men. Comfort ye men of little heart. Receive ye sick men. Be ye patient to all men. See ye that no man yield evil for evil to any man. But evermore sue [sow] ye that that is good, each to other and to all men."[72]

In this modern information age we are reminded that neither religious nor medical freedoms are consigned to the history books, and that the printed word (in whatever format) still matters. Today Wycliffe's Lollards have become China's "Shouters," so named because they urge "shouting" the gospel to their fellow Chinese. Men like forty-six-year-old Yu Zhudi have spent years in prison for distributing the Bible in their country.[73] Likewise, the issue of free and equal access to medical information has transformed itself from one of providing it in a language accessible to the people to one of providing cost-free, end-user access to full-text online medical research articles under the rubric of "open access." Culpeper resolved the former issue of access once and for all, but the latter is very far from settled and is now complicated by a morass of legal and economic concerns over copyright, proprietary control, and governmental responsibility versus private enterprise. These are not soon to be definitively resolved. Issues of equitable access to medical care are perennial topics on Capitol Hill as well, and while the issues seem to be continually muddied with politics, they are nevertheless as pertinent as in Culpeper's day.

While religious and medical freedoms then and now are circumscribed by very different specifics, the animating spirit between the "haves" and the "have-nots," between those in power and those seeking empowerment, is very similar. The book in your hands speaks to that spirit, and it is hoped that each reader will take from it his or her own inspirational message.

Yet readers need not have such lofty aspirations to enjoy *The English Physician.* Many of the recipes found herein were born of hoary traditions established by shadowy mystics and apocryphal ancients. The book brings to life the epic fantasy *Lord of the Rings* and the magical world of *Harry Potter,* with wizardry more wondrous than Gandalf's and potions more fantastic than those of Severus Snape. It conveys to the modern reader a time when astral positions and lunar phases were taken seriously, when plants were "signed by God" with shapes and colors suggesting their therapeutic properties, when mysterious "life forces" were revived with centipedes and mummy powder, when medicine was more sorcery than science.

Whether it is seen as an interesting medical first that transformed the American botanical and medical landscape or merely as a quaint literary excursion into a world long past, *The English Physician* has something for *every* reader. Culpeper would have approved of such a large audience.

Notes for the Introduction

1. Sometimes spelled Wyclif; the usage of *The Concise Dictionary of National Biography,* vol. 3 (New York: Oxford University Press, 1992), 3308, is preferred here.

2. Jonathan Hill, *The History of Christian Thought* (Downers Grove, IL: Intervarsity, 2003), 170–71.

3. W. R. Cooper, introduction to *The Wycliffe New Testament (1388),* ed. W. R. Cooper (London: British Library, 2002), vii.

4. For a thorough discussion of all the various Wycliffite Bibles, see Christopher de Hamel, *The Book: A History of the Bible,* (London: Phaidon, 2001), 166–89.

5. For a complete discussion of Culpeper's works and his printers, see Mary Rhinelander McCarl, "Publishing the Works of Nicholas Culpeper, Astrological

Herbalist and Translator of Latin Medical Works in Seventeenth-Century London," *Canadian Bulletin of Medical History* 13 (1996): 225–76. It should be noted that in Culpeper's original works he spelled the word "physitian," though bootleggers and later reprint editions opted for the more modern spelling of "physician."

6. Culpeper was not the first to call for an unveiling of medical secrecy. In 1632 Peter Levens, in his *Right Profitable Booke for All Disease,* asked rhetorically, "[W]hat reason is it that we should keepe secrete among a few, the thing that was made to be common to us al? . . . As for the knowledge of medicines, comfort of hearbes, maintenaunce of health, prosperitie of life, they be his [Christ's] benefits & proceed of him, to the end that we should in common helpe one another; and so to live together in his Lawes and commandments." Quoted in John B. Blake, "The Compleat Housewife," *Bulletin of the History of Medicine* 49 (1975): 33.

7. Barbara Griggs, *Green Pharmacy: The History and Evolution of Western Herbal Medicine,* 2nd ed. (Rochester, VT: Healing Arts, 1997), 109.

8. Quoted in Olav Thulesius, *Nicholas Culpeper: English Physician and Astrologer* (New York: St. Martin's, 1992), 68.

9. Quoted in Charles H. LaWall, *Four Thousand Years of Pharmacy: An Outline History of Pharmacy and Its Allied Sciences* (Philadelphia: J. B. Lippincott, 1927), 319.

10. Nicholas Culpeper, *The Complete Herbal* (1653; repr., Birmingham, UK: Imperial Chemicals (Pharmaceuticals), 1953), 407.

11. Ibid., 528.

12. Ibid., 408.

13. Quoted in Thulesius, *Nicholas Culpeper,* 67.

14. Benjamin Woolley, *Heal Thyself: Nicholas Culpeper and the Seventeenth-Century Struggle to Bring Medicine to the People* (New York: HarperCollins, 2004), 295.

15. McCarl, "Publishing the Works of Culpeper," 237.

16. Woolley, *Heal Thyself,* 295.

17. Oliver Wendell Holmes, "The Medical Profession in Massachusetts," in *Medical Essays, 1842–1882* (Boston: Houghton Mifflin, 1883), 342.

18. See comments in Fielding H. Garrison, *An Introduction to the History of Medicine,* 4th ed. (Philadelphia: W. B. Saunders, 1929), 289; Eleanour Sinclair Rohde, *The Old English Herbals* (1922; repr., New York: Dover, 1971), 163–70.

19. J. Worth Estes, "'To the Courteous and Well Willing Readers': Herbals and Their Audiences," *Watermark* 18, no. 3 (1995): 68.

20. David L. Cowen, *The Colonial and Revolutionary Heritage of Pharmacy in America* (Trenton: New Jersey Pharmaceutical Association; Madison, WI: American Institute of the History of Pharmacy, 1976), 7.

21. Patricia A. Watson, *The Angelical Conjunction: The Preacher-Physicians of Colonial New England* (Knoxville: University of Tennessee Press, 1991), 36.

22. See ibid., 76–77, table 3.1.

23. Ibid., 79.

24. George K. Smart, "Private Libraries in Colonial Virginia," *American Literature* 10, no .1 (1938): 40–41.

25. For a detailed discussion of the American botanical movement, see Alex Berman and Michael A. Flannery, *America's Botanico-Medical Movements: Vox Populi* (New York: Pharmaceutical Products, 2001).

26. John S. Haller Jr., *The People's Doctors: Samuel Thomson and the American Botanical Movement, 1790–1860* (Carbondale: Southern Illinois University Press, 2000), 47.

27. Alexander Wilder, *History of Medicine* (Augusta, ME: Maine Farmer, 1904), 706.

28. John Uri Lloyd, *Origin and History of All the Pharmacopeial Vegetable Drugs* (Cincinnati: Caxton, 1929), 373.

29. I was not the first to notice the Protestant connection; see John S. Haller Jr., *The Medical Protestants: The Eclectics in American Medicine, 1825–1939* (Carbondale: Southern Illinois University Press, 1994). Haller quotes Edward B. Foote, MD: "Eclecticism is as much a protest in the field of medicine as was Luther's Reformation in the domain of religion. We are protestants against the old dogmas of medicine, just as the disciples of Luther were protestants against the dogmas of the Papal church" (vii).

30. Wooster Beach, *American Practice of Medicine and Family Physician,* 10th ed. (New York: James McAlister, 1847), xiii–xiv. The emphasis is in the original.

31. Thulesius, *Nicholas Culpeper,* 107.

32. McCarl, "Publishing the Works of Culpeper," 226.

33. Thulesius, *Nicholas Culpeper,* 184.

34. F. N. L. Poynter, "Nicholas Culpeper and His Books," *Journal of the History of Medicine & Allied Sciences* 17 (January 1962): 160.

35. Woolley, *Heal Thyself,* 327.

36. Nicholas Culpeper, *Culpeper's Last Legacy* ([London]: N. Brooke, 1657).

37. Ibid., 48.

38. Woolley, *Heal Thyself*, 329–30.

39. Ibid., 326.

40. David L. Cowen, "The Boston Editions of Nicholas Culpeper," *Journal of the History of Medicine & Allied Sciences* 11 (April 1956): 156–65. See also John L. Thornton, *Medical Books, Libraries, and Collectors*, 2nd ed. (London: Andre Deutsch, 1966), 104; George E. Gifford, "Botanic Remedies in Colonial Massachusetts," in *Medicine in Colonial Massachusetts, 1620–1820* (Boston: Colonial Society of Massachusetts, 1980), 275, 263–88; Jeremy Norman, ed., *Morton's Medical Bibliography*, 5th ed. ([London]: Solar, 1991), 285, entry 1828.1; Thulesius, *Nicholas Culpeper*, 181.

41. Cowen, "The Boston Editions of Nicholas Culpeper," 157–58; Thulesius, *Nicholas Culpeper*, 181; McCarl, "Publishing the Works of Culpeper," 253.

42. George Emery Littlefield, *Early Boston Booksellers, 1642–1711* (1900; repr., New York: Burt Franklin, 1969), 12.

43. For details on the newspaper, see "The Boston News-Letter," information circular 5 (revised 1957), Library of Congress, Constituent Services, Serial & Government Publications Division. For details on Boone's first shop, see Littlefield, *Early Boston Booksellers*, 193.

44. Littlefield, *Early Boston Booksellers*, 93.

45. Ibid., 201.

46. Ibid., 199.

47. In 1700, for example, *The Compleat Gentlewoman and Chamber-Maid's Closet Newly Opened*, a book of domestic remedies, actually *re*opened an earlier work first issued in 1675 with a nearly complete verbatim reprinting of Hannah Woolley's *The Accomplish'd Ladies Delight*. See Blake, "The Compleat Housewife," 35–36.

48. A search performed September 15, 2005, in the Online Computer Library Center's (OCLC) WorldCat (the world's largest bibliographic database) and Research Libraries Information Network's (RLIN) Eureka (a high-end bibliographic database of the Research Libraries Group comprising many of the world's most prestigious research institutions) yielded the following holdings: the American Antiquarian Society, Duke University (copy incomplete with the last sixteen pages missing), Harvard University (formerly Boston Medical Library), the University of California, Los Angeles, and the University of Alabama at Birmingham.

49. Littlefield writes that "his shop and all of its contents were destroyed," *Early Boston Booksellers,* 196.

50. This ad ran in Boone's *Boston News-Letter.* For details see James Harvey Young, *The Toadstool Millionaires* (Princeton, NJ: Princeton University Press, 1961), 7–8. In combining book sales and proprietary medicines, Boone was following a common practice in England. For example, calculations of English sales outlets during the last ten years of Daffy's life (1674–84) reveal that merchants and booksellers topped the list, with physicians and apothecaries noticeably absent. See David Boyd Haycock and Patrick Wallis, *Quackery and Commerce in Seventeenth-Century London: The Proprietary Medicine Business of Anthony Daffy,* Medical History, supplement no. 25 (London: Wellcome Trust Centre for the History of Medicine, 2005), 19.

51. For additional particulars on this popular nostrum in an American context, see George B. Griffenhagen and James Harvey Young, "Old English Patent Medicines in America," *Pharmacy in History* 34 (1992): 205–6.

52. Figure from the online calculator "How Much Is That Worth Today?" Lawrence H. Officer, "Comparing the Purchasing Power of Money in Great Britain from 1264 to Any Other Year Including the Present," Economic History Services, 2001 <http://www.eh.net/hmit/ppowerbp/>.

53. Cowen, "The Boston Editions of Nicholas Culpeper," 157.

54. Anne F. McGrath, ed. *Bookman's Price Index: A Guide to the Values of Rare and Other Out of Print Books* (Detroit: Gale Group, 2002), 201.

55. McCarl, "Publishing the Works of Culpeper," 253.

56. Cowen, "The Boston Editions of Nicholas Culpeper," 157.

57. Ibid., 158.

58. For a detailed discussion of Galenic and Paracelsian theory, see Glenn Sonnedecker, *Kremers and Urdang's History of Pharmacy,* 4th ed. (1976; repr., Madison, WI: American Institute of the History of Pharmacy, 1986), 19–20 and 40–45 respectively.

59. Typical was the venerated physician/historian William Osler, who considered astrology in medicine largely a sophistry foisted upon an all-too-willing public. See his *Evolution of Modern Medicine: A Series of Lectures Delivered at Yale University on the Silliman Foundation in April, 1913* (New Haven, CT: Yale University Press, 1921), 119–25.

60. Poynter, "Culpeper and His Books," 157.

61. *Dictionary of Scientific Biography*, 8-vol. ed. (1981), s.v. "Delisle, Joseph-Nicolas."

62. See table 13 in J. Worth Estes, "Therapeutic Practice in Colonial New England," in *Medicine in Colonial Massachusetts*, 330–31.

63. Ibid., 346.

64. That climax was reached when Union surgeon William A. Hammond was tried and convicted of malfeasance on trumped-up charges. The *real* reason for his dismissal was that he removed two common mineral remedies from the U.S. Army Standard Supply Table (calomel and antimony). Leaders of the botanical medical movement had long argued that their counterparts in regular medicine were killing their patients with dangerous chemicals, calomel and antimony foremost among them. Thus, Hammond's act was interpreted by his colleagues as professional treason. Moreover, when it was discovered that numerous botanic physicians had (unbeknownst to the military) passed the medical exam for admission into the army medical corps and served with distinction, there was a heightened concern among regulars that they might actually lose their professional battle with these sectarians. Michael A. Flannery, "Trouble in Paradise: A Brief Review of Therapeutic Contention in America, 1790–1864," *Pharmacy in History* 41 (1999): 153–63; see also Michael A. Flannery, "Another House Divided: Union Medical Service and Sectarians during the Civil War," *Journal of the History of Medicine & Allied Sciences* 54 (October 1999): 478–510.

65. Orrin Hatch, *Square Peg: Confessions of a Citizen Senator* (New York: Basic Books, 2002), 82–84.

66. Ibid, 85.

67. Woolley, *Heal Thyself*, 351–52.

68. Rohde, *Old English Herbals*, 5.

69. Wilder, *History of Medicine*, 407–8.

70. Frederick F. Cartwright and Michael D. Biddiss, *Disease and History* (1972; repr., New York: Barnes & Noble, 1991), 49–50.

71. Daniel Defoe, *A Journal of the Plague Year* (London: E. Nutt, 1722), 276.

72. From 1 Thessalonians 5, in Cooper, *The Wycliffe New Testament (1388)*, 350.

73. See AsiaNews.it for March 9, 2004, "China Bible 'Smuggler' Released after 3 Years in Prison" <http://www.asianews.it/view.php?i =en&art=471>.

THE

English Physician.

CONTAINING,

Admirable and Approved

REMEDIES,

For several of the most usual

DISEASES.

Fitted to the meanest Capacity,

By *N. Culpepper,* Doctor of Physick.

Licensed, According to Order.

BOSTON,

Re-printed for Nicholas Boone,
at the Sign of the BIBLE, near
the Corner of *School-House-Lane.*
1708.

THE ENGLISH PHYSICIAN

To the Reader.

I have here made Publick to the World, some of my choicest Secrets in the Art of Physick, which I had once thought never to Publish; but the Importunities of the Publick Good, has so prevailed with me, above my private Interest, to serve my Age and Station in which I live. Be kind and good to your Poor Neighbour, for which you may expect the Blessing of God: And in so doing you will Compel me to Oblige the World with several other useful things, which I shall fit to the common Capacity of all People.

I am
Your Humble Servant,
N. Culpepper.

Aches, and Lameness in the Body, Joints, Limbs and Bones.

An approved Searcloth for all Aches.

Take Burgandy Pitch,[1] one Pound; White Virgin's Wax four Ounces; white Frankincense, two Ounces, powdered: Melt them all together in a Pipkin [small pot], stirring all well together; then pour out all into a Basin, or Pan of Water; then anoint thy Hands with Butter, and make thy Plaster, or Searcloth into Rolls.

---

1. More commonly today spelled Burgundy pitch, named after the spruce tree (*Pini burgundica*) from which it is obtained. This strong, pungent resin was believed to have regenerative properties and even to promote "benevolent energies."

An Excellent Ointment for the same.

Take the Gall of an Ox, White-wine Vinegar, Oil of Excester,[2] Aqua Vitæ [strong liquor], of each a like quantity, boil them gently on a Fire, keeping it scum'd, till it grow clammy, and with this bathe well the aching part, soaking it in well, by rubbing it in, before a Fire, with a warm Hand, Morning & Evening, still laying a Linnen Cloth upon it.

For Bone-ach, and the Gout.

Take of the best Aqua Vitæ, and Oil of Bays, of each a like quantity, mix them well together, and anoint the part well with a warm Hand before the Fire, and bind on it a Linnen Cloth, Morning and Evening.

For the Joint Ach, and the Gout, most Excellent.

Take the Juice of Sage, Aqua Vitæ, the Oil of Bays, Vinegar, Mustard, and of an Oxes Gall, of each a like quantity, put them all together in a large Ox Bladder. Tie it fast, and chase it up and down with your hand, during one hour & half, then keep it for your Use, & anoint the griev'd part Morning and Evening.

A Process against all Pains & Aches in the Back, Hips, Sides, Knees, or any part of the Body.

Take first Pil. Fœtida,[3] one drachm, to Purge now and then, and take them in Syrup of Roses; after Purging, procure Sweat thus.

---

2. Oil of Exeter was a popular polypharmacy concoction dating from medieval times. For a typical recipe see Paul Acker, "Texts from the Margin: Lydgate, Recipes, and Glosses in Bühler Ms 17," *Chaucer Review* 37, no. 1 (2002): 72. Culpeper's formula given in *Complete Herbal,* 522. Of this remedy he writes, "Many people by catching bruises when they are young, come to feel it when they are old: others by catching cold, catch a lameness in their limbs, to both which I commend this sovereign oil to bathe their grieved members with."

3. Sometimes called "stinking pill," this was made primarily of asafetida, a plant of the carrot family with such a bad odor that it was often referred to as "devil's dung," but also comprising some nineteen other ingredients. See J. Worth Estes, *Dictionary of Protopharmacology: Therapeutic Practices, 1700–1850* (Canton, MA: Science History, 1990), 84.

Take Guaiacum, one Ounce, Sarsaparilla, one Ounce and a half, the Root of Enulacampain,[4] one Ounce; boil them in a Pottle of small Ale, till half be consumed, then drink thereof a Quart in a Hot House, & Sweat often; Then in the House, bathe all the Body with this Oleaginous Balsome.

Oil of Amber, Oil of Turpentine, Oil of Foxes, Oil of Excester, and Oil of Chamomil, of each a like quantity, and mix it with some Brandy.

And if his Pains and Aches fall out to be most painful in the Night (as many times they do.)

Then at Night let him take this Potion, Syrup of Poppy, 3 Drachms; Syrup of Betony, one Drachm and a half; Waters of Bugloss[5] and Sage, of each an Ounce, mix them well together.

This Cured a Man Perfectly, when he was Lame all over his Body.

Take the Gall of an Heifer, for a Man; the Gall of a Steer for a Woman, Brandy, of each a like quantity, boil them together 'till it begin to be clammy, and before the Fire with a warm hand strongly bathe the Party Morning and Evening, till he be whole.

To heal and strengthen weak Limbs of Children, and those which cannot stand nor go. Most wonderful and Excellent to cure the Rickets.

Take Sage, sweet Marjoram, Rosemary, Time, Chamomile, Hyssop, Feverfew, Lavender, Balm, Mint, Wormwood, Rue, Winter Savory, and Bays of each a handful, beat them together to a Mass very well in a stone Mortar, then strain out the Juice and put it in a double Glass, the which stop well, and paste it all over with Dough, and set it in an Oven with Houshold Bread, and when it is drawn, break off all the Paste, and if the Juice be thick break the Glass, and put the Juice into a Gally-Pot [glazed earthenware jar]: And when you use it, take the quantity of 2 Spoonfuls of it, and put to it as much of the Marrow of an Ox Leg, melt them together, stir them well, and add to it a little Brandy;

---

4. *Inula helenium*, used as an expectorant, diuretic, cathartic, stomachic, and emmenagogue. Ibid., 78.

5. Buglossum. *Anchusa officinalis* was considered a "weak refrigerant." So-called refrigerants were cooling agents, somewhat analogous to an antipyretic. Ibid., 31.

and Morning and Evening anoint well before a Fire the Child's Arms, Sides, Thighs, Legs, Knees, Feet & Joints, bathing it well in with a warm Hand. Then give it some Syrup of Rhubarb (to open the Obstructions of the Liver) and mingle it with two ounces of Mint-water, mix it well, and give it the Child fasting. This will mightily strengthen the Limbs, and make the Child to stand & go. *Probat.* [*probatio,* a proven remedy]

APOPLEXY TO CURE.

Take of the best Aqua-vitæ well rectified from Phlegm one Pint, Oil of Vitriol[6] one Spoonful, mix them and let him drink thereof one Spoonful first in the Morning, and another last at Night.

Then let him Sweat in a Stove twice a week, and every time therein bathe him with Oleaginous Balsom. This is Excellent.

For the Joint-ach & Numbness.

Take six Spoonfuls of Dragon-water,[7] dissolve in it one drachm of Mithridate;[8] drink the same draught three Mornings together fasting, and sweat two Hours after it. This Cures.

AGUES AND FEVERS TO CURE.

A rare Secret to Cure all Agues whatsoever.

Take Venice Turpentine[9] half an Ounce; Incorporate it with as much Mastick of Sheep's Leather cut round, and lay it on the Navel pretty warm, a day before the Fit cometh, *Probat.*

---

6. Sulfuric acid. Diluted and used topically as a caustic and rubefacient (a so-called counterirritant), internally as an astringent, refrigerant, stomachic, or tonic. Ibid., 204–5.

7. A popular remedy during the period, perhaps containing *Arum maculatum* (dragon root). Its inclusion here is interesting for Culpeper writes, "I would not wish any, unless very well read in physic, to take them [the roots] inwardly" (*Complete Herbal,* 312).

8. A polypharmacy brew named after the first-century BC physician-king Mithridates. It contained around fifty different ingredients (opium among them). Culpeper gives its attributes, ibid., 476–77.

9. A balsamlike resin collected from larch trees.

Against an Ague.

Take a Pint of Milk, set it on the Fire, and when it boils put in a pint of Ale, take off the Curd, then put into it nine heads of Cardius [*Carduus Benedictus,* blessed thistle], then boil it till half be wasted, then to every quarter of a pint put in a good Spoonful of Wheat-flower, & a quarter of a Spoonful of gross Pepper, stir it well, and take that half Pint an Hour before the Fit cometh, and be sure to Sweat him in his Bed upon the taking of it.

A Plaister against an Ague.

Take a piece of Leather pricked full of Holes, spread it over with Venice Turpentine, and on that spread all over Rue and Frankincense, beaten into Powder, of each a like quantity, then bind it on the Wrist a little before the Fit cometh, and let it lie till the Fit be gone.

Against a Tertian Fever.

Take (at the coming of the cold Fit) half a pint of the distilled water of Germander: It helpeth assuredly; for Germander is styled by Physicians, the Scourge of a Fever.[10]

Against all burning and pestilential Fevers.

Take of the Herb Fluellin [an annual plant related to the snapdragon and foxglove] cut small, and infuse it 24 Hours in White-wine, then Distil it, and drink of this Distillation, with three Drops of Oil of Vitriol in every Draught, when he is thirsty. That hath cured Old and Young that took it.

An excellent Process of Cure of all Quotidian, Tertian, Quartane, Pestilential and Burning Fevers and Agues.

Take (at the first access, Purge the Patient with this Excellent Medicine) Aloes three drachms, Myrrh one Drachm; Saffron half a Drachm, Sugar Three

---

10. Culpeper writes, "The decoction [of germander] thereof taken for four days together, drives away and cures both tertian and quartan agues" (*Complete Herbal,* 118).

Drachms; and beat them well together, then infuse them in a Pint of White-wine over Night, and give it two several Mornings, half a Pint at a time.

His Drink a Julep.
And for his ordinary Drink, when he is Thirsty, let him use this Excellent Julep. Take White-wine Vinegar half a pint, Rose-water 1 pint, Conduit or Fountain-water [spring water], 1 pint; Seethe them together with a Pound of Sugar.

Phlebotomy.
If the Sick be high Couloured, then let him Blood as a chief Remedy; if no Spots appear in his Breast.

Sleep to Procure.
If he want Sleep, Take Syrup of white Poppy, one ounce; Distilled water of Lettice, two ounces, mix them and take it at Night, for Sleep cools the Body, and prevents motion, and Motion is one of the principal causes of heat.

Sore Mouth to Heal.
If the Mouth be sore, Take one Penny-worth of red Sage, grossly cut, on a handful of French Barley beaten, Roach Allom [alum?][11] one ounce: Boil all these together in a Pint and half of Springwater then dulcify it before it be cold with Honey, and therewith wash the Mouth, and gargle the Throat.

To make the Costive Laxative.
If he be Costive, make him Laxative with my Pilulæ Magistrales [Masterwort, a perennial resembling Angleica],[12] nothing comparable.

---

11. Probably a reference to alum drawn from a main source. The *Oxford English Dictionary* (*OED;* 12 vols. [1933; repr., Oxford: Clarendon Press, 1961]) defines roach as something mined from the main vein.

12. Culpeper writes: "Magistrantia, & c. Masterwort. Hot and dry in the third degree: it is good against poison, pestilence, corrupt and unwholesome air, helps windiness in the stomach, causeth an appetite to one's victuals" (*Complete Herbal,* 339).

His Diet.

His Diet must be Broths of Chickens, Knuckles of Mutton or Veal; but no Flesh, for that increaseth and feedeth the Fever.

Against a new Ague.

Take one drachm of pure Tobacco in the Leaf, infuse it all Night in half a pint of White-wine, then strain it and drink it, fasting two Hours after it. This will purge Phlegm and Choler throughly.

Against a burning Fever.

Take distilled Wall-nuts, a week or two before Mid-Summer, and give of that water one ounce and a half at a time, an Hour before the Fit. It Cures.

To keep the Belly open in a Feaver.

Take the Decoction of Prunes four ounces, wherein dissolve Manna[13] one ounce; then when they boil up, distrain them, and drink four ounces of the Liquor fasting.

An excellent Julep in all Feavers.

Take what quantity of Prunes you please, bruise them and distill them, and keep the Distillation in a great Glass, with a Tap in it at the bottom; then take four ounces of Prune-water, Juice of Oranges, Syrup of Gilli-flowers [gillyflower, any of several species resembling a pink carnation] two ounces, a few drops of Spirit of Vitriol; mix them, and let the Patient drink two or three spoonfuls at a time often.

Note, *That all Volatile Salts of Rue, Sage, Marjoram, Rosemary, and the like, being drunk in Wine, and Sweat upon it, cures all Feavers.* Van Helmont.[14]

To preserve your Juice of Oranges, buy your Oranges when they be cheap-

13. The resin of *Fraxinus ornus.* A mild demulcent cathartic that causes colic and flatulence. Estes, *Dictionary of Protopharmacology,* 123.

14. Jean Baptist van Helmont (1577–1644). A Flemish physician of the Paracelsian school famous for his discovery of carbonic acid.

est, & good store; then press out their Juice, then clarify it, and put it in a great Glass, that hath a Tap and Spicket in the bottom of it; then cover the Juice in the Glass one Inch thick with good sweet Sallet [salad] Oil; and so you may preserve your Juice as long as you will.

To strengthen the Heart in all Fevers mightily.

Take of the dryed Leaves of Marygold-flowers, beat them to powder, then take Turpentine and Rosin each a like quantity; then put them into an equal quantity of fine Hogs Lard, and incorporate them well together over the Fire, then spread thereof on a shield plaister of Leather, and lay it on the Breast over the Heart, and this will strengthen the heart unspeakably.

BLEEDING TO STOP IN ANY PART, INWARDLY, OR OUTWARDLY.

To stop the Bleeding at the Nose.

Take Bole Armoniack [bole armoniac, an Armenian clay used as an astringent], stamp it finely to Powder; then blow up some of it with a Quill into the Bleeding Nostril of the Patient, and it stops presently. *Probat.*

Against Pissing of Blood.

Take Sheep's Milk (highly praised herein above all) Fasting 4 ounces, mix with it a drachm of fine Bole Armoniack in Powder, & drink it up.

Against the Bloody Flux, and Pissing of Blood.

Take Conserve of Roses 1 ounce, Crocus Martis[15] 1 Scruple, mix them well, then take it on the point of a Knife in a Morning fasting, and do for three several Mornings together and be whole. *Probat.*

---

15. A combination of "purified iron filings" and sulphur; the mixture is heated and used as a deobstruent and emmenagogue. Ibid., 56. By the nineteenth century it was known in various permutations as Ferri subcarbonas (precipitated carbonate of iron) and Colcothar (calcinated sulphate "red oxide" of iron). See Robley Dunglison, *A Dictionary of Medical Science* (Philadelphia: Henry C. Lea, 1874), 233, 274, 414.

Against all Fluxes in Men and Women.

Take Syrup of Roses, and Syrup of Mints, 1 ounce of each, Bole Armoniack in Powder 1 Drachm, incorporate them in red Wine, make a Potion and drink it off.

To cool the Blood, Liver & Reins [kidneys].

Take Strawberry-Leaves, with the roots, what you will, boil them in white wine and Water, then strain them, & drink off the Decoction fasting, 1 pint.

Judgment on the colour of the Blood.

If the Blood come Wheyish, it comes from the weakness of the Reins.

If it come from fulness and largeness of Veins, then the party feels no pain.

If it come from breaking a Vein, then the Blood cometh more abundantly.

If it come by some sharp Humour gnawing the Veins, then the Blood comes by little and little, and the Reins are pained.

If the Blood appear red of Colour, and white Water flows with it, then the Blood is found.

If bubling Blood issue, the Stomach of the Party is Diseased.

If the Blood be green, then the Heart is grieved.

Against spitting of Blood.

Take Mastick and Olibanum,[16] in Powder, 2 Scruples of each, conserve of red Roses 2 Ounces, Diascordium[17] half an ounce; mix them together, & make an Electuary [a sweet medicinal candy], then take thereof Morning and Evening on the point of a knife, as much as a Nutmeg at a time.

16. Frankincense (the resin of *Bosellia carteri*) considered stimulant, diaphoretic, and cathartic. Estes, *Dictionary of Protopharmacology*, 141.

17. A preparation of opium invented by Girolamo Fracastoro in the early sixteenth century for use as a plague remedy. Ibid., 65.

Against Pissing of Blood.

Take the Juice of Purslain [*Trianthema monogynum*, a coarse fleshy weed],[18] make it into Pills with Gumtragacanth [a polysaccharide thickening agent, primarily of *Astragalis* spp.] and Gum Arabick, of each alike in Powder & take 5 Pills at a time. It helpeth.

To stop the Bleeding caused by Leeches.

Take a Bean, slit it in twain, take away the Skin, and lay it on a place where a Leech hath drawn, that bleedeth too much, and it will stop the bleeding.

Against spitting & vomiting of Blood.

Take of the Seed of St. John's Wort, with its Herb and Flowers, and boil them in White-wine, and drink of the Decoction (being strained) it helpeth, tho' it come by Bruises, Falls, breaking a Vein, or howsoever.

To expel Blood or Choler [bile] out of the Stomach.

Take 2 Drachms of the Seeds of St. John's Wort beaten into Powder, and drunk in a little Broth, doth gently perform it.

To stop Bleeding, or casting of Blood in a Consumption.

Take 3 Spoonfuls of the Juice of Sage, with a little Honey fasting, it presently doth stop it.[19]

Against the spitting of Blood with a Cough.

Take Bole Armoniack, Terra Sigillat [tablets made of earth], white and red Corral, of each half a Drachm, all powdered, Sugar of Roses half an ounce, stir them well together, with the white of an Egg, make a Looch [loch, a lambative or medicine made to be licked] thereof, & take a little often.

---

18. Culpeper considered purslain "of singular good use to cool the heat and sharpness of urine" (*Complete Herbal*, 206).

19. A close paraphrase of Culpeper, ibid., 228.

A Clyster against a sharp Humour, that issueth out Blood instead of Ordure [stool].

Take one pint and a half of new Milk, boil it to a pint with a handful of red Rose Leaves in it, then sweeten it with powdred Sugar, and give it up into the party, and let him keep it as long as he can.

BELLY INFIRMITIES TO CURE.

To reduce a hard Belly, and hard Sides.

Take Ungentum Dialthææ[20] 3 ounces, Ungent. Agrippæ,[21] oil of Chamomil, of each an ounce, incorporate them together with a little Brandy, and anoint the part Morning & Evening before the Fire, rubbing of it in strongly with a warm Hand, half an hour at a time.

Another for the same.

Take your own Urine, and drink a good Draught thereof Nine Mornings together. *Probat.*

Against the griping Torments and fretting of the Guts.

Take the Juice of Plantain clarified and drink it by it self, or in other Drink for divers days together, it wonderfully prevails, as aforefaid; as also, against all Distillations from the Head, and all manner of Fluxes in Men and Women.

Against Wind, & gripings in the Belly.

Take of the Roots of Kneeholm,[22] Anniseeds and Fennelseeds, half an ounce of each, make them all into Powder, and mix them well together with half an

---

20. An ointment made from althea, *Althea officinalis* or marshmallow. Estes, *Dictionary of Protopharmacology,* 62.

21. Also known as Unguentum Diabryonias. A mildly drawing ointment, possibly named for the early-sixteenth-century German physician Cornelius Heinrich Agrippa. Ibid., 4–5.

22. Also called butcher's broom, *Ruscus aculeatus.* According to Culpeper, it was "effectual in knitting and consolidating broken bones or parts of joint[s]." See M. Grieve, *A Modern Herbal,* 2 vols. (1931; repr., New York: Dover, 1971), 1:128.

ounce of Sugar, and take every Morning of it as much as will lye on a Shilling in Wine or Posset-Drink.[23]

Against the Griping in the Guts.

Take Salt of Wormwood half a Drachm, Andromachus Treacle[24] two Drachms, Conserve of red Roses what sufficeth to be made up into a Bolus,[25] and to be taken first in the Morning.

To Cure an extraordinary Flux of the Bowels.

Take 2 hard Yolks of Eggs, temper them with good Rose Vinegar, & give it to the Patient to eat first in the Morning. By this Medicine alone a Man was Cured of this Distemper, who had daily 70 Stools a day, when all other means failed.

Against Gripings & Wind in the Guts.

Take Oil of Ivy one Drachm in a Cup of Wine mixt, & drink it Fasting doth the Work.

---

23. *OED* defines as: "A drink composed of hot milk curdled with ale, wine, or other liquor, often with sugar, spices, or other ingredients."

24. A curious combination of terms, both of which refer to theriac or theriaclike preparations. Treacle was generally known as "Venice treacle," which contained opium and some fifty-seven other ingredients. Estes, *Dictionary of Protopharmacology,* 201–2. Theriac, also known as an Andromache after its alleged founder, Andromachus, was a similar polypharmacy nostrum. By the early eighteenth century the number and variety of recipes for this cure-all were legion. Ibid., 193–94.

25. Literally from the Greek *bolos,* meaning "lump." Culpeper does not give a definition even in his *Complete Herbal,* but they are generally considered simply large pills over five grains in weight. See Robert A. Buerki and Gregory J. Higby, "History of Dosage Forms and Basic Preparations," in *Encyclopedia of Pharmaceutical Technology,* ed. James Swarbrick and James C. Boylan (New York: Marcel Dekker, 1993), 7:303. A bit more vaguely, Culpeper's kindred domestic healer, William Buchan, defines a bolus thus: "They are generally composed of powders, with a proper quantity of syrup, conserve, or mucilage." See his *Domestic Medicine, or A Treatise on the Prevention and Cure of Diseases* (Fairhaven, [UK?]: James Lyon, 1798), 434.

A Clyster against pain and griping in the Bowels, Dysenteria.
Take Cows Milk 1 Pint, fresh Butter 1 Ounce, Gumtragacanth 1 Dram, the Yolks of 3 Eggs, Oil of Roses 2 Ounces; make it Blood warm, to the dissolving of the Gum, & so put it up.

BREATH, STINKING OR SHORT, TO CURE.

Against a stinking Breath.
Take a good quantity of Rosemary Leaves and Flowers, boil them in Whitewine, and with a little Cinnamon and Benjamin [the Benjamin tree or benzoin] beaten to Powder, being put therein, let the Patient wash the Mouth often therewith, and it will presently help. *Probat.*

Against shortness of Breath.
Take of Saffron in Powder 1 Scruple, of Musk in Powder 1 Grain, give them in Wine.

For the same.
Take sweet Marjoram and boil it well in Water, and drink of the Decoction first and last, and at other times. This helps all diseases of the Chest, & will make you breathe freely.

Against shortness of Breath with a Cough.
Take the Roots of Valerian and boil them with Liquorice, Raisins stoned, and Anniseeds, and drink of the Decoction often; this is singular good against the said Diseases, for it openeth the passages, and causeth the Phelgm to be spit out easily.[26]

Against a stinking Breath.
Take Myrrh, what you will, boil it in Water, and with the Decoction wash your Mouth often.

---

26. A paraphrase of the remedy given in Culpeper, *Complete Herbal,* 264.

BREASTS INFIRMITIES TO CURE.

A Pultess [poultice] for a sore Breast.

Take new Milk and grate white Bread into it, then take Mallows and red Rose Leaves, 1 handful of each, then chop them small, and boil them together till it be thick, then put in some Honey and Turpentine, mix them, then spread it on a Cloth, and apply it.[27]

For an Ague in the Breast.

Take good Aqua-vitæ and Linseed Oil and warm them together on a Chafing-Dish of Coals, dip therein 2 Cloths made fit for the Breasts, and lay them thereon as hot as may be suffered Morning and Evening.

Milk hard in the Breast to Cure.

Take Mint, Wallwort [perhaps walewort or dwarf elder] and Vervain,[28] of each a like, and with Hogs Grease stamp them together, and make a Pultess, and apply it.

To bring long and great Breasts to a little Proportion.

Take Hemlocks, shred them and boil them in White-wine, then make a Plaister of them, and apply them to the Breasts.

To Heal an Inflammation in the Breasts.

Take the whites of two Eggs, and two handfuls of Housleek,[29] let the Eggs be first well beaten, then stamp them both together and apply it.

27. Culpeper suggests many things for sore breasts (e.g., purslain, quince, figs) but none of the ingredients listed here.

28. Probably not the tropical varieties of vervain but rather vervain sage or *Salvia Verbenaca*. Culpeper's belief that this plant "scatters congealed blood" makes the application here to breast milk obvious. See Grieve, *A Modern Herbal*, 1:205.

29. A housleek, *Sempervivum tectorum* (sometimes called commonly hens-and-chickens). Now an adventive plant in America. Merritt Lyndon Fernald, *Gray's Manual of Botany* (1950; repr., Portland, OR: Dioscorides, 1987), 734.

If Milk Curd in the Breast, to Cure.

Take Gumtragacanth and Gum Arabick, of each a like, dissolve them in Rose-water, then put to the Mucilage the whites of raw Eggs, and Oil of Violets; compound all well together, then make a plaister thereof, and apply it.

To heal Ulcers in the Breast, altho' very grievous.

Take Oil of Sulphur & touch them, then make this Ointment; Take the Yolks of new Eggs, 2 ounces, Turpentine, Butter, Barley Flower, & Honey of Roses half an ounce of each; Incorporate them all in a Mortar, & therewith dress them till they be whole.

BACK INFIRMITIES TO CURE.

Against Pains in the Back, and coldness and weakness in the Reins, and want of an Appetite to a Woman.

Take Parsnip Roots, as many as you please, let them be fair and great, cut away the tops, then put them into an Earthen Pot with water, and double the Roots in Sugar, then boil them with a slow Fire till they be tender, then take them out and lay them on a Grid-Iron to cool, then pair them & take out their Piths [pits], and then put them into a new Earthen Pot glazed, put to them as much clarified Honey as will cover them, and boil them till the Honey do throughly penetrate them; then take them from the Fire, and put to them two parts of Cloves, and one part of Cinnamon and Ginder [ginger], then bray them with the Roots together, and being well mixed, take thereof fasting one Ounce at a time, and you will find a marvellous Effect.

Against Pain in the Back and Reins. This hath helped many grievously affected.

Take a new laid Egg, beat it well in a Porringer [shallow cup or bowl with a handle]; then take four Spoonfuls of White-wine, and two Spoonfuls of red Rose-water, one Penny-worth of Sugar-candy in powder, mix them well with the beaten Egg, and drink it up fasting: as much at Night will not hurt you.

To Strengthen the Back, and to take away pains and aches there.

Take Paracelsus's plaister,[30] Melilot [leaves and flowers of sweet clover] plaister, Diapalma,[31] Diachylon,[32] and plaister of Minium [lead oxide] of each a like, incorporate them together over the Fire, make a plaister on Sheep's Leather, and apply to the Reins & Back.

To strengthen a weak Back.

Take Nep [catmint, *Nepeta catavia*], Clare [clary, a species of *Salvia*], and the Pith [spinal cord] of an Ox-back, chop them very small together; then take the Yolks of 3 new laid Eggs, beat them well, then strain them, and try them together, then eat it fasting & drink a draught of Sack [white wine imported from Spain and the Canary Islands] after it. Use this six or seven times together.

BRUISES, HURTS, CONGEALED BLOOD TO CURE.

To take away black & blue Spots, coming of stripes and bruises.

Take Rheubarb and boil it in Wine, and bathe the part, or anoint the place with Oil, wherein Rheubarb hath been boiled.

A Powder against falls, & inward bruises.

Take Bole Armoniack, Dragon's Blood,[33] and Mummy;[34] Two Drachms of Each; Sperma Cœti [whale oil] One Drachm, Rheubarb Half a Drachm; make them all into Powder, and give half a Drachm or more at a time in Wine.

30. Perhaps opodeldoc, a word applied by Paracelsus to certain plasters for which he was particularly known. These plasters were made from an alcoholic solution of soap, camphor, essential oils, and laudanum. Estes, *Dictionary of Protopharmacology,* 143.

31. A dessicating plaster made from palm, white lead, olive oil, and water. Ibid., 63.

32. A simple variation on the former without the palm. Ibid., 61.

33. *Sanguis Dragonis,* a flammable gum resin from fruits of the *Daemonorops propinquus* and *D. ruber.* It gets its name from the deep red color obtained when placed in alcoholic solution. An astringent and incrassating tonic (one that purportedly thickens bodily fluids). Ibid., 171.

34. Powdered Egyptian mummy in an alcoholic or other suspension medium was considered a restorative tonic. Ibid., 131–32.

For all sorts of bruises and hurts in any part of the Body.

Take the Leaves of Bugle [*Ajuga reptans*], Scabious [any herb of the genus *Scabiosa*], and Sanicle,[35] of each a like quantity, bruise them and boil them in Hog's Grease, until the Herbs be dry, then strain all into a Pot, and stop it up close. It is of singular use to cure all hurts in the Body, if anointed therewith.

Against all Bruises, Hurts, Wounds and Inflammations.

Take *Paracelsus* Plaster half an Ounce, Diapalma as much, green Melilot one quarter of an Ounce; incorporate them over the Fire, make Plaisters o' it and apply it. This is good also against all Inflammations coming of heat.

The Vertue of Paracelsus's Styptick Plaister.

Its Vertues are great & excellent; It keeps back the concourse and falling down of Humours; it dries superfluous Mixture, it will expel Wind, it cures a Bruise or Ache, it heals Wounds and Ulcers, breeding nothing but found Flesh; it defends from Putrefaction, and will keep free from Corruption forty Years.

For black and blue Spots and Cricks in the Neck.

Take Mustard-seed, powder it well, then mix it with Honey, and apply, or make the Powder up in Wax and apply it. This is good also against the crick in the Neck by Cold.

BURNINGS AND SCALDINGS TO CURE.

Against burning with Gunpowder.

Take the whites of Eggs, and stamp and beat them well together; then wet a Linnen Cloth in the liquid Matter, and lay it thereon where it is burned, and still wet the Cloth therewith on the outside thereof, that it may not remain dry, and this will fetch out the Fire and heal. *Probat.*

---

35. *Sanicula* (common name black snakeroot), allegedly derived from *sanare,* "to heal." This herb was used as an astringent. See Fernald, *Gray's Manual,* 1088 and Estes, *Dictionary of Protopharmacology,* 172.

For a Burn.

Take Castile Soap, put it in a melting Pan over the Fire, and stir it 'till be as thick as a Salve, then make Plasters thereof, and lay on the burnt place.

To heal a Burning or Scald without any Scar.

Take Sallet Oil, well beaten in fair Water, or Unguent Populeon,[36] and therewith anoint the Burned or Scalded place three days twice a day, and it will fetch out the Fire.

Then take the inner Bark of Elder, Hart's Tongue [hound's tongue][37] and Housleek, of each four Drachms, Sheep's Trickles [?] one Handfull, Sheep's Suet four Drachms, boil them together to a good thickness, and put thereto Wax 1 Drachm, then strain it, and Plaster-wise apply it to the Grief, twice a Day 'till it be whole, without Scar.

Another for the same.

Take of the Juice of Plantain, Housleek, and the lesser Comfrey,[38] of each four Ounces, of Sheep's Dung (dissolved in the said Juices) 2 Ounces, Sheeps Suet 1 Pound shred, then boil them together over a gentle Fire to a due height, then strain it, and reserve it for your Use.

Against Burning and Blasting, by Gunpowder, or Lightning.

Take of the Juice of Purslain, and mingle it with as much Oil of Roses, and anoint the part therewith, Morning and Evening.

To Cure Burning and Scalding.

36. Popular ointment made from poplar, opium leaves, mandrake, and other botanicals. Estes, *Dictionary of Protopharmacology,* 155.

37. "Hart's tongue" is probably an error since Culpeper recommended it largely for "hardness and stoppings of the spleen and liver" (*Complete Herbal,* 125). Culpeper considered hound's tongue (*Cynoglossum officinale*) good for scalds and burns, 138–39.

38. Probably common comfrey, *Symphytum officinale.* Although found in America today, it was naturalized from Europe. Fernald, *Gray's Manual,* 1199.

Take the Ointment of white Lillies, and anoint the part first, and then Morning and Evening apply the said Ointment Plaister-wise.

Baldness to help.
And this will bedeck a bald Head, or other part with Hair.

Another.
Take the Distilled Water of the Sperm of Frogs, and bathe the part well, letting it dry of it self, and then lay Clouts wet therein on it.

BITINGS BY MAD DOGS, SERPENTS, &C.

For the Biting of a Mad Dog.
Take of Gentian Root[39] in Powder one Drachm, and give in Carduus Water [holy water]. Or,

Take Gentian Root in Powder 30 Grains, of Rue in Powder, 1 Scruple, of Pepper, powdered 5 Grains. Give it in Angelicæ Water.

Against the Bitings of Serpents, and of a Mad Dog.
Take Agrimony,[40] boil it in Wine, & drink the Decoction for Serpents; and for a Mad Dog take the Leaves of Agrimony, bruise them and bind them to the bitten place.

Against the Biting of an Adder or Viper.
Take 1 Drachm of the tops of the Stalks and Flowers of great Century, beat them into Powder, and drink them in Wine. This is a very good help.

---

39. Gentians number about 180 species, and the reference here could be to *Gentiana lutea* (yellow gentian), *Swertia perennis* or, more likely, *Gentianella anglica*. Culpeper believed that English gentians "have been proved by the experience of divers physicians not to be a whit inferior in virtue to that which comes from beyond the sea." See Grieve, *A Modern Herbal*, 1:347–49; Culpeper quote cited on p. 349.

40. *Agrimonia Eupatoria*. Although found from Massachusetts to Wisconsin and Minnesota, it is adventive from Europe. Fernald, *Gray's Manual*, 867.

Against the Stinging of Bees & Wasps.

Take of the Leaves of Marsh-mallows,[41] bruise them, or rub them on the place, and it will take away the pains, redness, and swelling.

CORDIALS.

An Excellent Cordial.

Take the Flowers of Marygolds, and lay them in Brandy, till the Tincture be fully taken out, then pour it out from the Flowers, and over a few Coals vapour away the Tincture, till it come to be thick like an Electuary.

A Cordial against Wind in the Stomach, or any other part.

Take 6 Spoonfuls of Pennyrial-water [pennyroyal, a perennial mint], and put thereto 4 drops of the Oil of Cinnamon, mix them, and drink it any time, Fasting two hours after.[42]

A Cordial for the Head & Stomach.

Take a preserved Nutmeg, and cut it in Four Quarters; and eat One Quarter of it at Breakfast, and another in the Afternoon. This is very good.

A Cordial to be taken at Sea, and good any where else.

Take Syrup of Clove Gilly-flowers one ounce, Confectio Alkermes[43] one Drachm, Borrage water[44] one ounce & a half, of Mint-water as much, of Mr.

41. Another likely botanical introduction from Europe via Culpeper, *Althaea officinalis* is common from Connecticut to Virginia westward to Michigan and Arkansas. The root of this perennial yields a natural mucilaginous paste. Ibid., 1002.

42. Interestingly, Culpeper was careful to distinguish the pennyroyal mint from other kinds of mint and does not include it among his recommendations for "wind" in his herbal, and nowhere does he suggest cinnamon for this problem.

43. A confection made from kermes, once thought to be a berry of an evergreen oak but, in fact, a pregnant insect (*Coccus ilicis*). Used in making scarlet dye, it was also considered mildly astringent and a tonic (especially for the heart). Estes, *Dictionary of Protopharmacology*, 109–10.

44. *Borrago officinalis*, considered tonic, aperient, and diaphoretic. Ibid., 30.

Mountford's Water,[45] or other hot Cordial Spirit as much, and as much Cinnamon Water; temper all these together, and take a Spoonful at a time, when you see cause.

Two Cordials to be taken in a Burning Fever.

Take a quarter of a pint of Mace Ale,[46] sweeten it with half an ounce of Syrup of Gilly-flowers, and give it to Drink in their Burning Fit.

Or,

Take the Juice of an Orange, and as much red Rose Water, mix them and sweeten them with White Sugar Candy: These will refresh the Spirit, and Cool and Allay their Drought.

COUGHS [47] AND SHORT BREATHINGS.

For a Cough of the Lungs.

Take Green Box[48] dried, powdered fine, and take of it as much as will lie on a Groat [an old British coin] at a time in White-wine warmed, first and last, till you be well, which will be when you see your self spit Blood, then leave your Medicine for you are well. *Probat.*

---

45. Moundeford's "Aqua Cordialis" appeared in the 1618 edition of the *Pharmacopoeia Londinensis.* It consists (among other things) of angelica, blessed thistle, and licorice. *Pharmacopoeia Londinensis of 1618,* with an introduction by George Urdang (1618; repr., Madison: State Historical Society of Wisconsin, 1944), 103. The inclusion of "Mr. Mountford's Water" here is interesting since it is not in Culpeper's *London Dispensatory* (1653).

46. Mace appears ten times in *The English Physician.* An old English herb similar to tansy, also called costmary. Culpeper also referred to it as "Balsam Herb." Frequently used to give a spicy flavor to ale, its pleasant odor gave it a variety of uses, from relieving headache to helping stomach disorders. See Grieve, *A Modern Herbal,* 1:226.

47. Many of the remedies here appear to be artful "additions" to Culpeper since he recommends only angelica, garlic, and horehound for coughs.

48. Perhaps a reference to wintergreen, also known as boxberry. Grieve notes its use as an astringent and aromatic. *A Modern Herbal,* 2:849.

Another for the same.

Take 1 pint of pure English Honey, set it over warm Embers in a new glazed Pipkin, that holds a little more than a Pint, and as the Scum or Froth riseth scum it; then take 2 ounces of red Currants and put it into the Honey, and let them simmer together a good while; then put to them two ounces of Powder of Liquorice, as much of Anniseeds in Powder, one ounce of pulveriz'd Elecampane,[49] and incorporate them well together. Then take of it first in the Morning, at Four in the Afternoon, & last at Night, the quantity of a Nutmeg at every time.

For a Cough.

Take Sallet Oil, Aqua vitæ, and Sack an equal quantity of each, beat them well together, and before the Fire rub the Soles of your Feet with it.

An Electuary against a Cough.

Take of pure honey 4 ounces, Powder of Elicampane 2 drachms, powder of liquorice 1 drachm: mix them, & take thereof on the point of a knife often.

For a Cough coming of a thin Rheum.

Take Mastich and Olibanum in Powder, of each 2 Scruples, Conserve of red Roses 2 Ounces, Diascordium half an Ounce, mix them, and take thereof first and last the quantity of a Nutmeg.

For a Chin Cough.

Take a handful of Rue, stamp it and mingle it with English Honey, and make a Conserve; give of it first and last, and at other times, the quantity of a Damson[50] at a time.

---

49. *Inula campana,* an expectorant, diuretic, diaphoretic, cathartic, stomachic, and emmenagogue. Estes, *Dictionary of Protopharmacology,* 78.

50. A tall shrub or small tree, also known as bullace or *Prunus insititia.* Another introduction from Europe. Having escaped cultivation, today it is naturalized in thickets and borders of American woods. Fernald, *Gray's Manual,* 876.

For an extream Cold or Cough.

Take Hyssop Water 6 Ounces, red Poppy Water 4 Ounces, 6 Dates, 10 Figgs, slice them small, 1 handfull of Raisins of the Sun stoned, the weight of a Shilling of the Powder of Liquorice; put these into the said Waters, then let them stand 5 or 6 Hours upon warm Embers, close covered, but not Boil; then strain it forth, and put in as much Sugar of Roses as will sweeten it: Drink of this first and last, and at 4 in the Afternoon, four Ounces at a time.

Against a Cough and Distillation of thin Rheum.

Take Olibanum in Powder, and mix it with Conserve of Roses, and first and last, and oftner if need be, take the quantity of a Nutmeg on the point of a Knife at a time.

Against a Cough, Wheezings, Distillations, and Shortness of Breath.

Take of Wood Betony [*Pedicularis spp.*] in Powder, mix it with pure Honey, and take it as in the last Receipt before is specified. It is available.

Another for the same, most Excellent.

Take Hyssop and Rue of each a like quantity; cut them and boil them in white Wine; then dulcifie the Decoction with Honey, & take a Draught of it first and last, and oftner if need be. It is excellent.

For a Chin Cough.

Take wild Thyme, boil it in white Wine, and drink of the Decoction often, and first and last. A better Remedy for this Infirmity scarce grows.

For a perillous Cough.

Take Sage, Rue, Pepper, and Cummin; of each of the Herbs a like quantity, and seeth them together in white Wine; dulcifie the Decoction with Honey, and take thereof first and last, and oftner if need be, 1 Spoonfull at a time.

Consumption.

Against a Consumption.
Take Rice beaten to Powder, and sifted clean from the Husk, then seeth it in Milk of a Red Cow, then season it with Sugar, and a little Cinnamon and Mace; then take a few blanched sweet Almonds, and stamp them, then strain them into the Milk; the eating a Breakfast of this cures a Consumption, & helps Conception.

Another, and which restoreth Nature lost.
Take good Malmsey [a Madeira wine], or Malaga [wine from Malaga, Spain] 1 Pottle, put in it as much Crum of white Bread, hot out of the Oven, as will suck up all the Wine; add thereto of Cinnamon powdered 4 Drachms, and 10 Cloves bruised, then distil them in *Balneo Mariæ;* then add to what is come over, so much Sugar as will fit your Taste, with 2 grains of Musk. The Dose is Three Spoonfuls first and last.

For a Consumption, a Distillation, and to restore Strength.
Take Rose-water 3 Pints, Old Malaga 3 Pints, new Milk 1 Pottle, gross Pepper 1 Ounce, Cinnamon 2 Ounces, of sliced white Bread 1 or 2 Penny Loaves, the Yolks of 12 new laid Eggs beaten, or more, of Sugar 1 Pound: Distil all these so long as any Water will come; take of this Water (with a little Pepper) a Draught fasting, and you will find much good by it.

For a Consumption and Cough of the Lungs.
Take new Milk of a red Cow two Quarts, a quantity of Shell-snails, taken out of their shells, what sufficeth, Flower of Sulphur half an Ounce, or less, the Yolks of 4 new laid Eggs beaten; boil them well together, then strain it, and dulcifie it, and Eat thereof first and last.

Another for the same.
Take Benjamin in Powder, as much as will lye on a Groat, as much Flower of Brimstone [sulphur], the Yolk of a new laid Egg, one spoonful of red Rose

Water, brown Sugar Candy, as much as a Wallnut in Powder, mix them, and take this Dose in the Morning Fasting, and Fast 2 Hours after it. Do thus nine mornings together & be whole.

An Excellent Remedy against a Consumption.

Take a Pottle of Rose-water, or Goat's or Asses Milk, or the Milk of a Cow all of one Colour (in want of the other) and put therein only the Yolks of Fifty Hen's Eggs, new laid, beat the Yolks, and mix them well with the Milk and Rose-water; then Distil them, and give of the Water Distilled to the Patient, first and last warm, with a Cake or two made of Gold & Perls. This is Excellent.

For a Consumption, and Cough of the Lungs.

Take one Pound of the best Honey, dissolve it in a Pipkin; then take it off the Fire, & put into it two Pennyworth of Flower of Brimstone, as much of Powder of Elicampane, as much of Powder Liquorice, two Penny-worth of red Rose-water; then stir them well together, and put it in a Gally Pot close stopped: Take as much thereof at a time, as half a Wall-nut, first and last, and at any time in the Day or Night when the Cough troubles you, and let it melt down your Throat by degrees.

To restore a weakned Person by Sickness, & to preserve from a Consumption.

Take 3 Pints of good new Milk, and put thereto 1 Pint of red Wine, with the Yolks of 24 Hens Eggs, new laid, beaten together; then put in as much fine white Bread, as shall suck up the Milk and Wine; then Distil it with a soft Fire, and take a Spoonful of this Water in your Pottage or Drink; and this in one Month will prevent the Consumption.

For a Consumption.

Take a Breast of fat Pork, boil it in red Cow's Milk, and drink thereof a good Draught first and last, and at 4 in the Afternoon.

Against a Consumption, and to restore a decayed Nature.
Take Goat's Milk one Quart, Rice beaten and sifted four Ounces, Sugar one
Ounce, the Flesh of Dates, one Ounce, Beef Marrow two Spoonfuls, Cinna-
mon half an Ounce; Boil them all together, and Eat thereof Morning and
Evening.

CONVULSION AND CRAMP.

Cramp to cure.
Take Brimstone and Vervain, beat them together, and bind them on the Pulse,
and be ever freed.

Against convulsions in Old & Young.
Take Thirty Piony [peony] Berries, husk them, then make them into Powder,
and drink off as much as will lie on a Sixpence at a time in white Wine, first
and last.

Against the cramp & shrinking of sinews.
Take one handful of Chick-weed, 1 handful of dried red Rose Leaves (but not
distilled) boil them in a Quart of Muskadine [wine], till a fourth part be consumed; then put to them a Pint of Sheep's-foot Oil,[51] then let them boil a
good while, still stirring them well; then strain it out, and anoint the part
warm before the Fire, with a warm Hand, This (by God's Blessng) helps in
three Dressings.

Pills against the Convulsion.
Take Opopanax,[52] Rue, Serapinum, Pepper, of the Juice of Lovage, Myrrh, of

---

51. Probably similar to neat's foot oil, made from the hooves of cattle.

52. Its usage is unclear here. Perhaps it is opopanewort, marsh woundwort. Grieve notes its
use among a number of herbalists of the period. *A Modern Herbal,* 2:862–63. Also it might very
well be a reference to *Pastinaca Altissima,* used as late as the nineteenth century as an antispasmot-
ic. See Dunglison, *Dictionary of Medical Science,* 765. (See also note 84.)

each 1 Drachm; Powder what is to be powdered, and with the Juice of Cowslips, make it into a Mass for Pills. The Dose is a Drachm every second or third Night, if need require.

For the Cramp.
Take the Philosopher's Oil of Tiles,[53] and anoint the part therewith by the Fire: It quickly penetrateth, and is a Soveraign Remedy against the Cramp, Gout, *&c.*

Oil of Rue doth the like.

Another.
Take of Juniper Berries fasting every Morning, they heat and rift the Cramp, & keep the Body in Health.

CANKER.[54]

For a Canker in the Breast, or elsewhere.
Take Pulverized Antimony, and convey it into it, it will kill it.

To cure a Canker or Soreness in the Mouth most wonderful.
Take Penny-royal, red Sage, red Fennel, Rosemary Tops & Mints, of each a good handful, half a handful of Hyssop: Shred them, and boil them in a quart of white Wine, and thereto put the quantity of 2 Wall-nuts of Roach Allom, and as much Honey as will make it sweet; then strain it through a fine Cloth, and wash and gargle the Mouth well, for it will cure it.

For the Canker in the Mouth or Nose.
Take the green Leaves of Holly, and burn them to Ashes; then mix them with

---

53. Later sold as British oil, philosopher's oil was comprised of liquid exuded from heating powdered bricks or tiles that had been soaked in rosemary oil. In 1742 Michael and Thomas Betton patented their "Oil of Bricks," a similar liniment touted as a remedy for rheumatism and scurvy. Estes, *Dictionary of Protopharmacology,* 30–31.

54. None of the following resembles Culpeper's remedies for canker.

half so much of the Powder of Burnt Allom, and blow it with a Quill into the grieved part, and it will Cure Man, Child, or Beast.

Corns and Warts.

To Destroy Corns.
Take of a Cow's Gall, and wet thy Corns therewith often, and let them dry of themselves; it will pluck them up by the Roots.

A Plaster to take away Corns.
Take Galbanum,[55] Ammoniacum,[56] of each alike; dissolve them in Vinegar of Squills [*Urginia maritima*, or sea onion], then boil them to a just consistency, adding a few drops of Oil of Vitriol; then spread it on Leather, and apply it to the Corn.

Against Warts.
Take Water of Agrimony, make it sower [sour] as Vinegar with Oil of Vitriol; and wash your Warts therewith, and they will fall out without pain.

For Warts and Corns.
Take fair Water half a Pint, Mercurius Sublimate[57] 1 Penny-worth, Allom as much as a Bean; boil all together in a double Glass in Water, till a Spoonful be wasted, and rub them therewith, always warming it before you use it.

55. Gum resin of *Ferula galbaniflua*. Applied externally, it allegedly disbursed swellings and ameliorated skin abrasions and similar conditions. It was also thought to draw out pus and thus promote healing. Estes, *Dictionary of Protopharmacology*, 87.

56. Extract of *Dorema ammoniacum* (gum ammoniac). Applied externally, its properties were similar to those of galbanum but also a soothing emollient.

57. Also known as *hydrargyrus muriatus corrosivus*, or corrosive sublimate (mercuric chloride). A common topical for skin inflammations, though very dangerous in unskilled hands. Estes, *Dictionary of Protopharmacology*, 99.

To take away Warts.
Take Shell-snails, prick them, and with the Juice that comes from them rub thy Warts every Day, for seven or eight Days together, and it will destroy them.

CHILDRENS INFIRMITIES TO CURE.

To prevent the Falling Sickness, and Convulsions.
Take of red Coral in powder 10 Grains, give it in Breast Milk to a new Born Child, for the first Food it takes after its Birth. It mightily strengthens the Brain.

To make them Teeth easily.
Take pure Capon's Grease well clarified, as much as a Nutmeg; twice as much Honey, then mix them together; three or four times in a day anoint the Gums when they are Teething.

Against Agues and Fevers, coming by pain in breeding of Teeth, or otherwise.
Take one spoonful of Ungent Populeon, two spoonfuls of Oil of Roses, mix them, then before the Fire anoint the Child's bowing places of his Arms, Legs, soles of its Feet, Fore-head and Temples, twice a Day, chafing it well in with a warm Hand.

Against Wind and Phlegm.
Take Sugar-candy in Powder, and in Saxifrage-water give it in a Spoon often.

Against the Worms.
Take Myrrh and Aloes of each alike, finely powdered; and with a few drops of Chemical Oil of Wormwood, or Savin [actually sabin, leaves of *Juniperus Sabina*], with a little Turpentine, mix them, and make them up for a Plaister for the Childs Navel.

For a Thrush, or sore Mouth.

Take an empty Egg-shell, by sucking the meat out at a hole on the top, then fill the Shell with Honey and burnt Allom mix together, let it boil on the Fire, still stirring it with a Bodkin, and dress it.

A Clyster for a Child, or for a Woman with Child, very safe.

Take a pint of new Milk, put in it 3 Ounces of Sugar-candy, boil it well, and being a little cool, put it up into the Body.

Against the Cough in Children.

Take 1 Ounce of Hog's Grease, half an Ounce of Garlick, bruise and stamp them together, and anoint the Soles of the Feet at Night warm, & then bind a Plaister thereof on the Soles.

Against the sticking out of the Navel.

Take the Juice of Purslain, and mingle it with as much Oil of Roses, mix them, and wet Clothes therein, and bind them on the Navel.

A Purge for tender Children.

Take a quantity of Liquorice, Anniseeds, small Raisins, and a handful of Hyssop, slice the Liquorice, beat the Seeds, shred the Hyssop, and boil them all in white Wine; then strain it, and give of it in a Spoon or otherwise, from half an Ounce to an Ounce, or more at a time.

COLICK.

For the Colick.

Take of the Electuary of Bayberries [*Myricacea* (wax myrtle) family] one Drachm, Oil of Amber 6 drops, Oil of Anniseed 8 drops, Oil of Vitriol half a Scruple: mix them, and make a Bolus, take it in a Wafer wet in water on the point of a Knife.

Against the Wind-Colick and Stone.

Take Electuarium Reginæ Coloniens.[58] Is an excellent Remedy against the Colick and Stone: the Dose is a Drachm taken every Morning, which is commended as a Jewel.

Against the Colick.

Take Castoreum one Drachm in a Cup of sweet Wine, or in 3 Ciathes [cyath, little cup] of Aqua Mulsa [honey water]. This is exceeding good Fasting, or often in Beer.

Another.

Take of Manna one ounce, Oil of sweet Almonds two Ounces; dissolve the Manna in Oil, and give it.
Note, Manna must not be boiled, but dissolved and strained.

Against the Colick and Stone.

Take a Cup of Wormwood Wine Fasting; it is an excellent Preservative against the Colick and Stone, and to walk much, but sit little.

Against the Colick & Iliack Passion.

Take a Load-stone, and lay it to the Navel, & presently the Grief will cease.

An Electuary for the same.

Take the best Treacle one ounce, Castoreum, Long Pepper, of each one ounce and half, Opium one Scruple: mix them exactly into an Electuary.

---

58. A complex polypharmacy electuary that contains, among other things, seeds of saxifrage, liquorice, caraway, anise, fennel, parsley, carrots, acorn, cumin, juniper, bayberry, valerian, ginger, goat's blood, sugar, in white wine. A paraphrase of *Complete Herbal,* 491–92.

CLYSTERS.

A Clyster to Purge Choler and Phlegm.
Take a pint of Milk, brown Sugar three Ounces, a little Salt, whereof make a Clyster, and with a Pipe put it into the Body.

This must be given not too hot, nor too cold, about Four of the Clock in the Afternoon, and two Hours after drink a Draught of Mace Ale.

Take a pint of Milk, make it into clear Posset-Drink with a Quart of Beer; then take off the Curd; then put in the Posset-Drink, Anniseed, and sweet Fennel-feed, of each 2 Ounces; boil these to half a Pint or more, then strain it out hard, and dissolve in it 2 Ounces of brown Sugar Candy, and a little Bay-Salt, with two Spoonfuls of Oil Olive, & put it up.

Another.
Take a pint of new Milk, making it scalding hot, then take it from the Fire, and put into it the Yolk of a new laid Egg beaten, with 2 Ounces of brown Candy, or brown Sugar, and put it up Blood warm.

To heal the Ulcerations and Flux of the Guts.
Take the Juice of Purslain, and put it up into the Fundament [anus] with a Clyster-Pipe.

DROPSIE.

Against the Dropsie, an Ointment.
Take Ungentum Artanitæ Mesue [?], and Ungentum Agrippæ,[59] of each alike, mix them well, then anoint the Belly twice a Day: If you anoint the Stomach, it will cause to Vomit, if the Belly then it Purgeth by Stool, and emptieth the Belly of much Water.

---

59. Briony roots, wild cucumbers, squills, orris root, dwarf Elder, etc., steeped seven days, boiled, and then made into an ointment with oil and wax. Ibid., 532.

Note, That before every anointing, you must rub the Belly well with a dry Cloth that is pretty course.

An Excellent Drink for the Dropsie.
Take one Pottle of white Rhenish Wine [wine from the Rhine], Cinnamon beaten one Ounce, one Pint of green Broom Ashes; put them together in an Earthen Bottle 48 Hours, stir them often, then drain them thro' a piece of Cotton twice, then drink of it one quarter of a pint cold in the Morning, another 1 Hour before Dinner, another 1 Hour before Supper, and another when you go to Bed. Usually 1 Pottle heals, if not, use more.

Another.
Take the inner rind of Elder, and boil it well in sweet Wort [sweet malt water], then drink half a pint thereof Fasting, it cures. *Probat.*

An Excellent Purge against the Dropsie.
And every third or fourth Day Purge the party with your usual Purge in Conserve of Roses.

EARS, NOISE AND DEAFNESS.

Against Noise and Singing in the Ears.
Take the Juice of Summer Savory, heat it, and mix with it a little Oil of Roses, or of Amber, and drop thereof into the Ears warm.

Another for the same.
Take a Clove of Garlick, peel it, make two or three holes through, and fasten it to the end of a thread, then dip it in fine English Honey, and so put it into the Ear, and stop it in with black Wooll, and lye on the other side; let it lie in 7 or 8 Days, you may pull it out by the Thread.

Another for the same, very excellent.
Take Oil of Castor, Oil of Roses, Oil of sweet Almonds, of each 1 Ounce;

mingle them with a little quantity of Aqua Vitæ, boil them to the Consumption of the Aqua Vitæ, and put 3 or 4 drops in the Ear to Bed-ward, and stop it with Cotton and a grain of Musk.

To get an Ear-wig, or other Worm out of the Ear.

Take the Juice of Wormwood Rue, and Southernwood [a bushy shrub, *Artemesia abrotanum*], of each alike, mingle them well, whereof put some into the Ear, and bind a Plaster of the said stamped Herbs to the Ear. This will kill it in five Nights.

Or,

Take a piece of an old Apple, and bind it into the Ear all Night, and lye on the same side all Night, and in the Morning quickly pull out the Apple, and the Worm will come with it.

EVIL DIGESTION TO CURE.

To help Concoction.

Take common Salt one ounce and a half, Pepper six Drachms, Cummin-seed half an ounce, Caraway-seed, Cinnamon, Zedoary [white tumeric, *Curcuma zedoaria*], of each 3 Drachms, Ginger and Mace of each 2 Drachms and a half; powder them, & mixt, eat it as Salt with your meat.

To help Digestion.

Take half a drachm of the dryed Root of Lovage [a Mediterranean plant, *Levisticum officinale*], in fine Powder in wine often; it doth wonderfully warm a cold Stomach, helpeth Digestion, and consumes superfluous Moisture there, easeth inward Gripings, expelleth Wind, & resisteth Infection.

An excellent help to Digestion.

Take Mustard-seed and Cinnamon one drachm of each, beat them together into fine Powder, then add half as much of Mastich in powder, and with Gum Arabick dissolved in Rose water, make them up into Troches of about half a drachm weight a piece, and eat one of them 1 Hour or 2 before meals. *Let Old People make much of this Medicine.*

Eyes Sore, to Cure.

To take away all spots in the Eyes, and superfluous Water.
Take of clear Antimony two grains, red Rose water 3 ounces, mix them together, and let them stand 24 Hours, then drop 4 or 5 drops of the clearest into the Eyes twice a day.

A Powder to preserve the Sight.
Take Eye-bright, Betony, of each 1 handful, Mace and Fennel-seeds, of each 2 drachms, make them into Powder, and give thereof at a time half a drachm first & last, in Broth or Beer.

A Jerusalem Colerium [collyrium, a topical for the eyes] for sore red Eyes, which Itch and Burn.
Take Tutia Alexandriæ [zinc oxide] 1 ounce, beat it into fine powder, then mingle it with 1 quart of white Wine, and put thereto dryed Roses 1 ounce, boil it with a soaking Fire, till half be wasted, then strain it into a Glass, and stop it close, and Morning and Evening drop some in your Eye. But Purge the Head first.

Pills to Purge the Head and Eyes of Rheum.
Take Extractum Rudij[60] 1 Scruple, Resin of Jalop 4 grains, Oil of Guaicum 2 drops; make them into Pills, and take them at once.

A water to heal all manner of sore Eyes.
Take Fennel, Vervain, Roses, Celandine, and Rue, of each 2 ounces: distil them, and wash thy Eyes therewith twice a Day.

60. A reference to *pilule Rudii,* a cathartic containing aloes and colocynthis. It likely received its name from Rudius, a small town in southern Italy. Estes, *Dictionary of Protopharmacology,* 168.

To clear the Sight very well.

Take Rose Water in a Saucer, then take clean Myrrh the quantity of a Nut, bring it into powder, then tie it in a Linnen Cloth that is clean, and let it lie in the Rose-water Twelve Hours, then with a Feather wash thy Eyes therewith twice a Day. *Probat.*

To keep back the Humour that flows to the Eyes and Teeth.

Take Mastich and Frankincense in fine Powder, of each alike, make them up into a Plaister, with white Wine and the white of Eggs; lay it to the Temples.

An excellent Collyrium for sore Eyes.

Take old white Wine 1 pint, white Rose-water 4 ounces, Tutia Alexandriæ 1 drachm; mix these and strain it, then beat the Whites of roasted Eggs in a Mortar, then pour the Wine and Rose-water on them, then strain it out hard, keep it close, and wash with a Feather twice a Day.

For a Weft⁶¹ of the Eye-lid, that darkens the Sight.

Take the Juice of Fenel, and wash it therewith, and drop thereof 3 drops into the Eye, twice a day. It will take away the Weft immediately, and restore the sight.

An excellent Water to Cure all Griefs in the Eyes whatsoever.

Take of unflaked Lime 3 Ounces, infuse it in a pint of Rain Water in a Jar Glass 3 days; stir them well together, then let them settle 24 Hours, then Cant off the clear very clean, add thereto the whitest Sal Ammoniack, powdred very finely 10 drachms; let it dissolve therein by standing and by stirring often, then let it settle, and filtre it, drop 3 drops of this into thy Eye at a time, Morning, Noon, and Night, till you be well. This cureth all Spots, Perls, Webs, Films, Cankers, Burnings, or any thing else in the Eye.

To destroy a Pin and Web in the Eye.

Take of Spirit of Vitriol 1 drop, drop it into the white of an Egg hard roasted,

---

61. *OED* defines as: "A film over the eye [cataract]."

and it will turn it into Water of which water drop into thine Eyes Morning, Noon, and at Night.

To heal all sorts of Sore Eyes.

Take the Herb Bucks-horn Plantain, a quantity, bruise it and boil it in Ale or Wine, and drink thereof for some Mornings and Evenings together, a Draught; it stoppeth all Distillations, and helpeth.

To cure the Obstructions of the Optick Nerves.

Take the true Herb Valerian, seethe it in Wine, then strain it, and let the Patient drink of it as his common Drink 3 or 4 Months together.

The best Remedy for Redness of the Eyes.

Take white Vitriol, make it very pure by often dissolutions and coagulations, 1 drachm; then dissolve it in Rain water 10 ounces, then filtre it divers times thro' brown Paper, then add to it 1 scruple of common Salt.

For a Pin, Web, or Perl in the Eye.

Take white Ginger, and grind it to Powder on a Whet-stone into a fair Bason, and add to it as much Salt as the Powder, then grind them well together in the Bason, and temper them with white Wine; then let them stand 24 Hours, then cant off the thin part that lies above into a Glass, stop it, and going to Bed, with a Feather wash thy Eyes, and be whole.

A precious Pill against all Fluxes of the Eyes.

Take the Leaves of Senna, of Turbith, of each 2 Drachms, Pil sine quibus esse nolo[62] 3 Drachms, Fenel-seed 2 Drachms; powder them, mix them and with

---

62. Literally, "pills I do not wish to be without." The specific reference here is to Culpeper's contemporary Robert Burton, in his *Anatomy of Melancholy* (1628; repr., London: Chatto & Windus, 1907), 444, in which he quotes Mesue as desribing *Hiera* as "*Pilulæ sine quibus esse nolo.*" Mesue was referring to *Hiera picra* (a noxious plant sometimes called "hicry-picry"), but in the context here it most likely is a reference to *Pilulæ sine Quibus,* a complex preparation of aloes, scammony, and assorted ingredients. See *Complete Herbal,* 498.

Syrup of Fumitory, or of Apples make a Mass; the Dose is a Drachm, till you be whole.

FALLING SICKNESS.

Against the Falling Sickness.
Take of the best rectified Aqua Vitæ, without Phlegm, one pint, Oil of Vitriol 1 Spoonful, mix them well together, and let the Patient drink thereof first & last, and he shall be holpen, altho' he have had it 10 Years, and fell every Hour.

Another.
Take that part of a Woman's Skull, that groweth on the hinder part of the Head (it is whiter than the rest of the Skull) beat it very fine to powder, and give the party as much as a Pea at a time in Syrup of Violets.

To raise one that is fallen quickly.
Take of Rue and Wormwood of each a handful, and make them into a mixt Powder together, and blow some of it by a Quill into the Nose of the party that doth fall, and he will rise presently.

To cure the Falling Sickness.
Take the Roots of Male Peony, for a Man (and the Roots of Female Peony for a Woman)[63] wash them clean, then stamp them somewhat small, and put it in Sack to infuse 24 Hours at the least; then strain it and drink a good draught thereof first and last, for sundry days together, next before and after the Full of the Moon.

Against the Falling Evil.
Take single Peony Seeds and beat them in a Mortar to powder, take as much

---

63. As late as the early twentieth century, botanic physicians still touted peony as a "minor nerve sedative." According to Finley Ellingwood, a prominent professor of Eclectic medicine, it was "soothing to the nervous system" and "curative wherever there is irregular muscular action." See his *American Materia Medica, Therapeutics, and Pharmacognosy* (1919; repr., Sandy, OR: Eclectic Medical, 1998), 129–30.

of it as will lie on a Shilling, in 3 or 4 spoonfuls of black Cherry Water, before & after the Full of the Moon, for divers days together Fasting.

Another that will not fail, good for Women.

Take the Roots of Peony beaten to powder, 1 drachm in Wine, Ale, or Broth, given in a Morning some days before and after the Full of the Moon, it Cures the Falling Sickness, if not too far spent; for it drives away all passions from the Brain, Heart and Spleen: also it helps the windiness of the matrix, suffocation of the Mother, & stopping of the Courses; & will give easie Deliverance to Women in Labour.

FISTULAES.

A perfect way to Cure a Fistula.

Take Alum 2 Pound, as much of white Copperas, beat them to a fine Powder, then put it into an Earthen Pan, let them dissolve to Water over a quick Fire, then take 6 ounces of Verdigrease [copper acetate], 4 drachms of white Mercury, both made into fine powder, then put them into the former water, stir them well together, and let them boil to a Stone, then beat it into powder, and mix with it 6 ounces of Bole Ammoniack made into fine powder, which keep in a Box for your use. Then take a gallon of Smith's oldest Water, let it boil in a Kettle, and shake in as much of the said powder by little and little, as will lye 6 times on a Shilling, let it boil a walm [gushing point] or two, then take it from the Fire and let it settle, then pour the clearest into a Glass, or Bottle, and keep it for use; And that is, to pour out as much of the Water as will wet two Cloths three or four times double, and lay them one after another all over the place grieved hot, wringing them first to prevent the running about of the Water. Do thus with clean Cloths twice a day, the Water stains and poisons that which drinks it in. This is an absolute Cure of the Fistula, and never fails.

To Cure Fistulaes, and old Sores, and Cankers, most admirably.

Take Oil of Vitriol 1 ounce, put it to 3 pound of Saturn [lead] filed into 5 parts, and let it be all eaten with the oil of Vitriol by degrees, one part after another, and when you have a good quantity of it, put it into a Retort, and put in with it 1 pint of white Wine, and distil it in Sand twice from the Fæces, and your Medicine is perfect.

This is excellent.

To Cure a Callous Fistula.
Take of the Root of black Hellebore,[64] bring it to powder, and leave of it in a callous Fistula, two or three days together, it will consume it quite.

A Drink to Cure the Fistula.
Take Valerian, Tormentil [*Potentilla Tormentilla*], Clove-gilly flowers, red Beets, red Chickweed, Pellitory of the Wall,[65] Galanga [*Alpinia officinarum*, or China root], Zedoary, Bay-berries, of each a like quantity, boil them all in white Wine, then strain it, and give of the decoction first and last, four spoonfuls at a time.

Fluxes.

Note, *Venice Treacle is good against all Fluxes of the Belly.*[66]

For the Flux, a pleasant Medicine.
Take Sallet Oil half a pint, Nutmegs beaten half an ounce, Cinnamon in powder 1 ounce, Mace one quarter of an ounce, fine Sugar half a pound; mingle these together, and eat of it 3 or 4 times a day. This hath Cured many.

64. *Helleboris niger*, also known as Melampode. Culpeper was probably also familiar with *H. Fœtidus* and *H. Viridus*, both of which are common substitutes for *H. niger*. Grieve, *A Modern Herbal*, 1:388; *Complete Herbal*, 131–32.

65. A curious redundancy since *Parietaria* (Pellitory spp.) is derived from the Latin *paries*, or wall, the habitat of the original species. Fernald, *Gray's Manual*, 559.

66. Culpeper gives the formula for this complex polypharmacy preparation, *Complete Herbal*, 478. For Culpeper it was a virtual cure-all: "It resists poison, and the bitings of venomous beasts, inveterate headaches, vertigo, deafness, the falling sickness, astonishment, apoplexies, dulness of sight, want of voice, asthmaes, old and new coughs, such as spit or vomit of blood, such as can hardly spit or breathe, coldness of the stomach, wind, the cholic, and iliac passion, the yellow jaundice, hardness of the spleen, stone in the reins and bladder, [etc.]."

An excellent Potion against all sorts of Fluxes.
Take Syrup of Roses and Syrup of Mints, of each 1 ounce, of Bole Ammoniack 1 drachm; incorporate them together, and with some red Wine make a potion. This also is good too against many Reds and Whites [diarrhea] in Women.

A perfect Cure of the Bloody Flux.
Take Conserve of Roses 1 ounce, Crocus Martis 1 scruple; mix them well together, and take it on the point of a Knife first in the Morning, and Last 2 Hours after. It cures tho' it hath been of a long continuance. *Probatum.*

Against the Flux Diarrhoea and Dysenteria.
Take every third day at a time 10 grains of Crocus Martis in Juice of Sloes of the Wood:
  This is a most Excellent Medicine.

Another for the Dysenteria.
Take 20 Yolks of boiled Eggs, Nutmegs beaten to powder, 2 ounces, red Wine 2 quarts; let them infuse one Night, then distil them in *Balneo* according to Art: The Dose is 2 ounces Fasting.

A Plaister of great use.
Take Bole Ammoniack, Dragon's Blood half a drachm of each, Mastich 1 drachm, Myrrh half a drachm, Venice Turpentine 3 drachms; beat what is to be beaten into fine powder and with Rosin and Wax what sufficeth, make them all into a plaister, and lay it upon the Navel and Belly.

French Pox.

If Buboes appear, then let him not Blood by any means. But no Buboes appearing, then let him Blood in the beginning in the Vein called Hepatica *in the right Arm. Then empty the Body by degrees of all the Evil Venemous & Malicious Humours, for which none are better than Extractum Rudij in Pills, or Mercurius*

Dulcis[67] *proportionably made up in the said Extractum; will do far better: But if that do not succeed, then if necessity require, you must empty the Humours by Fluxing.*

Pills to Flux in the Cure of the French Disease.

Take Sagepenum [gum resin of sagaen, *Ferula persica*] dissolved in white Wine 2 ounces, Salt of Guaicum,[68] Colocynthis,[69] Diagridij,[70] of each of them 1 ounce, Turbith Minerale[71] 10 drachms, Musk 1 scruple, Oil of July-flowers 12 grains; make them into a Majs; the dose is from 12 to 20 grains, for ten days together in the morning, or until the Patient sufficiently doth Flux at the Mouth.

If his Throat or Mouth be sore, to Cure.

Take one penny worth of red Sage, French Barley two handfuls, Roch Allom in Powder 2 Ounces, with Mint and roses half a handful of each, boil them all in one quart of water, then strain it, and while it is hot dulcify the Colature [strained mixture] with honey: with this warmed, wash, gargle, and serringe the Mouth & Throat 2 or 3 times a day.

If Puses, Scabs and Sores break out, heal with this Ointment.

Take Ungent Egyptiacum[72] 1 ounce, mingle it with one drachm of Mercurius

---

67. This is the same as calomel (mercurous chloride), the most popular of all the mercurials after 1595. See Estes, *Dictionary of Protopharmacology*, 34.

68. According to Grieve, *Guaiacum officinal* "obtained a great reputation about the sixteenth century, when it was brought into notice as a cure for syphilis and other diseases" (*A Modern Herbal*, 1:380).

69. Colocynth, or *Citrullus colocynthus* (bitter apple). A powerful cathartic, known to be lethal at more than a teaspoonful of the powder, yet the key ingredient in *Pilula Colocynthidis, Exstractum Colocynthidid Compositum*, etc. Ibid., 1:50.

70. Probably diagredium or scammonium. The gum resin of scammony, *Convulvulus scammoniua*, a strong cathartic. Dosage was crucial and could be fatal in unskilled hands. Estes, *Dictionary of Protopharmacology*, 174.

71. *Turpeth mineralis,* a mercurial devised by Paracelsian chemist Dr. Oswald Croll in the sixteenth century. Ibid., 197.

72. "Egyptian ointment," made of copper acetate, vinegar, and honey; used as a soughing agent. Ibid., 72–73. Interestingly, Culpeper writes, "It cleanses filthy ulcers and fistulas forcibly, and not without pain, it takes away dead and proud flesh, and dries" (*Complete Herbal*, 525).

Sublimate, and anoint therewith and if it smart beyond Suffering, then take Plantain water, Fumitory water, and Rose water; of each alike, mingle them, & touch the smarting part with it, and it will asswage the Pain.

If Nodes, or Knobs, or Wheals [pustules] appear, then use this.

Take Plantain and Rose Waters of each 1 pint, roch Allom and Sublimate of each 2 drachms, bray the two last into powder, put them together into a pipkin, boil them till half the water be consumed, then let it settle, and cane off the clear into a glass: and when you use it, mingle some of it with a tripple portion of plantain and rose water together, and then touch them therewith: And if they be on the face then first anoint them with Oil of Scorpions, or the fat of a Hen.

To preserve the Nose.

Take waters of Rose, violet and plantain, of each alike, a little wine Vinegar, Roch Allom in Powder a little, and a little honey, dissolve them over the Fire, and let the Patient snuff up strongly into the Nose; this cures and heals.

If the Teeth be loose, fasten them with this.

Take Plantain water, mix it with Oil of Sulphur, and touch therewith the Gums, and after they be mundified [cleansed], wash well thy Teeth and Gums with thy lotion aforesaid.

If a Bubo appear in the Groin, cure it thus.

Take Emplastr Paracels, diachylon Magnum, flos Ungentorum, Diachylon cum gummi, Emplastr. Mucilaginis, Emplistrum de Melilot of each alike, then incorporate them together, over a gentle fire, then make plaisters on sheeps Leather, and apply it to the Bubo morning and evening warm.[73]

And when it is broken, use the same plaister, only add to it in the melting

---

73. Perhaps the most complex recipe of the entire book. A combination of plaster of Paracelsus, flower of ointments, *Diachylon Magnum, Diachylon magnum cum Gummi,* a plaster of mussilages, and a plaster of Melilot mixed together. For plaster of Paracelsus, see note 30. The others are given in Culpeper, *Complete Herbal,* 544–48.

more of Flos Ungentorum and Emplastrum Betonicæ [plaster of betony][74] more than the rest, and that will draw it and heal it.

Now when all the evil humours are prepared, purged and emptied, you must come to your diet drink.

The first simple Decoction.

Take (in Winter) one Pound and a half of Guaicum 18 pints of Water; but in Summer (when it will not keep so long) Guaicum 6 ounces, and water 6 Pints, in both which the wood must be infused 12 hours or more. Let the water for the infusion be warm, almost seething hot, and keep the pot close stopped, let the decoction boil till half be wasted: so much for the first Decoction: always remembring, to save the Scum or Froth, for that is good to anoint the Pustules & Scabs.

To make the second Decoction.

Take the same wood without infusing any more, and boil it again in the same quantity of Water to the consumption of a third part.

The quantity of these is to be taken according to the strength of the party from 4 ounces to 8 ounces; and in a Child from 4 ounces to 6 ounces, and not exceeding 10 ounces then the disease is most rebellious, and always must be taken very hot, and sleep upon it if you can.

The first Decoction you must take first and last and the second Decoction, at and between Meals: some take this Decoction 30 days, some 40, some 60 days, to make the more surer Cure.

Their Meat must be roasted dry at Noon, and their Supper must be sweet Almonds, Raisins of the Sun stoned, and fine Bisket, or Bread made of the finest Flower.

And let him forbear Venery as he tenders his Life, and all chafing, fretting, and impatiency, for that inflames the Blood, stirs up Cholerick Humours, and is a great Enemy to the Cure.

---

74. For details see ibid., 540.

Note, In this Sickness, let the patient beware of taking cold: And beware of Costiveness.

Against the Falling of the Fundament.

Take Ungent, sumach,[75] when the fundament is fallen, anoint it therewith, then put it up and it will out no more.

Others for the same.

You may do the like with Bole Ammoniack, and with Dragon's Blood, and with Myrrh every one by themselves, brought into fine Powder.

Another for the same.

Take Olibanum in Powder, & strew it on the tuell [anus] fallen down, and then put it up.

FACE.

To Cure a Swelled Face.

Take wild Crabs, gathered on Midsummer-day, and distilled in a Limbeck, and with the distilled Water of them, wash thy Face often, and the intent will follow. *Probatum.*

To take away Spots, Morphew,[76] Freckles, and Sun-burning from the Face, Neck, Arms and Hands.

Take of the Juice of Lemmons 2 ounces, Rose-water, Mercurius sublimate in powder, 2 Drachms, ceruss [actually, ceruse or white lead] in Powder 2 Drachms; put it all together, then add to it Borax 2 Drachms, Camphire 1 Drachm, both in Powder; mix them well together into an ointment, with

75. A complex preparation of sumac, galls, myrtle berries, acorn cups, cypress nuts, etc. that Culpeper calls "a gallant drying and binding ointment . . . if the fundament fall out, when you have put it up again anoint it with this ointment, and it will fall out no more" (ibid., 536).

76. The *OED* defines as a leprous or scurfy (scaly) eruption.

which anoint your Face going to Bed, and let it dry on. And in the morning, wash thy Face with Butter and Rose-water mingled together. *Probat.*

A rare Secret to preserve the Beauty of the Face, Neck, Hands, Arms, &c.

Take Spanish Wine 9 times distilled, to every Quart put 2 ounces and half of sweet Benjamin in Powder; it is made in 12 Hours thus: Wash your Bottles clean, and let them be well dried; put in your Wine and Benjamin, and for 2 or 3 Hours shake them well together, then let it settle, and so use it thus; put a Spoonful or two of it into a Bason of fair water, and it will turn it like Milk, with which wash; for it is the most excellent thing in the world to the purposes aforesaid, and for the rareness of the Secret, is commonly sold for 20 *s.* a Pint.

For a white Scurf, or Pimples in the Face.

Take a Pint of white wine Vinegar dissolve in it 1 ounce of Camphire, of Roch Allom one quarter of an ounce, and a little Bay Salt, and let them stand together well stopped in a Glass, 14 days, then wash the part therewith.

For a red Face.

Take the distilled water of Cucumbers; it cureth the reddest Face that is, if often washed therewith.[77]

Gout.

A marvellous Remedy to Cure the Gout, it never fails.

Take half a pound of unwrought Wax, as much of Rosin, Labdanum[78] 1 ounce, Litharge [?][79] of Gold Four Ounces, White Lead in Powder and searfed

---

77. Culpeper writes, "The face being washed with their juice cleanses the skin" (*Complete Herbal,* 86).

78. The *OED* defines as a soft, dark, and fragrant oleoresin made from rockroses (*Cistus*) often used in perfumes.

79. Litharge typically means white lead, so its usage here seems unclear. White gold perhaps?

[served] 12 Ounces, then take a pint of Neats-foot Oil, and set it over a Fire in a pot, and mingle it with the Wax and Rosin, and when it is melted, put in all the other Powders, then stir it with a Stick as fast as you can, until dropping a Drop into a Saucer it appear hard, then take it from the Fire, anoint some clean, even Board, with Neats-foot Oil, and as soon as you can handle it for heat, make it up into Roles, and with Plasters of Leather made thereof, apply it to the part grieved Morning and Evening, and if it remove, follow it with your Plasters till it be quite gone.

An excellent Remedy against the Gout and the Dropsie.

Take Extractum Catholicon,[80] Pil Hermodac,[81] Pil. Arthritic[82] of each three scruples, mix them well and make them into Pills as big as a little Pea; take thereof at a time 5 Pills, three mornings together, about three or four of the Clock in the morning. It cures.

To Cure the Gout perfectly.

Take quick Lime, what you will, quench it in running Water, and then stir it about, till it be like a Hasty-pudding, then spread of it Plaster-wayes upon a Cloth, and apply it to the part grieved, only one Plaster to a grieved part and no more, and lay on your Plaster as hot as the Patient can suffer it. Colour your Lime with Saunders,[83] or Bole Ammoniack, or Dragon's Blood, that it may not be known.

Against Pain in the Gout.

Take Aqua vitæ 4 drachms, Sage 1 ounce, Opium 1 drachm, Saffron half a

80. Regarded as a cure-all, usually an electuary that "purged the humors." Estes, *Dictionary of Protopharmacology,* 42.

81. Perhaps pills of Hermodactils. For details see Culpeper, *Complete Herbal,* 495.

82. A complex preparation of *Iris tuberosa,* Indian spice, ginger, and ten other ingredients. See the *Pharmacopoeia Londinensis of 1618,* 186.

83. There were two types known: *Santalum Citrinum* (interior wood of yellow sandalwood or yellow sanders, *Santalum album*) and Santalum Rubrum (interior wood of red sanders, *Pterocarpus santonicum*). Estes, *Dictionary of Protopharmacology,* 172.

drachm, Camphire half a drachm, Oil of Foxes 2 Ounces, let all these be well mixed, & make a liniment, & anoint the grieved part, this is very Sovereign.

Against the hot and cold Gout.

Take Garlick and Houseleek of each alike quantity, stamp them very well together, till they be like a salve, and plaster-wise apply on a Cloth.

To ease any kind of Gout.

Take Opopanax[84] and puls [?] of raisins of the Sun of each alike quantity, easeth any kind of Gout being applyed plaster wise to it.

A sovereign Ointment against the Gout.

Take Oil of Bays, Aqua vitæ, Juice of Sage, Vinegar Mustard, and Ox gall of each alike quantity, put them into a Bladder, that is far too big to hold them and tie them up close, then chafe them up and down with your Hands one hour and half together; then have you as good an Ointment for the Gout as the World can afford.

Another for the same.

Take the herb Sparagus [asparagus] and stamp it very well, & then fill a walnut shell full of it stamped, and apply it to the place pained, bind it on, and in six or eight Hours, it will draw a blister, then which cut, and let out the water then take a Colwort-leaf, and lay to it, till the Malady be remedied.

Note, *The flower Crowfoot will do the like, so Canthrades* and *Leven* [leaven, yeast].

For all sorts of Gouts.

Take 1 drachm of the Electuary Catholicon going to Bed, and in the Morning drink a good draught of warm posset-drink, and then go about your affairs, it helps Gouts of all sorts.

---

84. A gum resin from *Opopanax chironium* considered a gentle cathartic, deobstruent, antispasmodic, and emmenagogue. Ibid., 143. (See also note 52.)

Another.

Take dwarf Elder, mingled with Bull's suet and stamped into a plaister, it is a present remedy for the Gout.

GREEN-SICKNESS.[85]

To Cure the Green-Sickness.

First cleanse the Body by gentle Vomits, then by Purges, or both together: Then
Take of Steel in fine powder 1 ounce, fine Sugar beaten small 5 ounces, Mace, Cloves, and Cinnamon, of each 1 Drachm, dry the Sugar & Spices very well by the Fire, then beat them to powder and keep them very dry by the Fire in a Box, that the Steel may not rust, & keep them well mixt; then take every day Fasting a good spoonful of it dry, and Walk One Hour or more upon it.

Against the Green-Sickness.

Take of Nutmegs pounded half a pound, put to them 1 quart of Sack, 1 pint of Water of Sloes,[86] boil this in a clear Decoction close, then strain it, and put to this Liquor, Cinnamon one Ounce, rinds of Pomegranates one ounce, Mace 1 drachm; boil it again close, then strain it hard, and give it Fasting 3 spoonfuls warm. And it will Cure.

Another for the same.

Take one quart of white Wine, 2 handfuls of Marygold Flowers, Pennyrial red Mints, of each one handful, stamp them small, and put the Wine to them, with a Penny-worth of Saffron, then strain it (it must not be boiled) and put it in a Glass close stopped, and let the Party drink thereof (only Luke-warm) 4 days together, and let the Patient use vehement Exercise, and abstain from rest and sleep in the day time.

---

85. Today this disease is known as hypochromic anemia or iron deficiency. See J. Starobinski, "Chlorosis—The 'Green Sickness,'" *Psychological Medicine* 11, no. 3 (August 1981): 459–68.

86. Probably the European sloe, *Prunophora spinosa* (an Old World plum). See Fernald, *Gray's Manual,* 876.

Another for the same.

Take an Orange, and cut off the top of it, then take out a little of the meat; then put therein a little Saffron and clap on the top and roast it gently, and when it is roasted put it presently into a pint of white Wine; keep it very close covered, and drink 4 ounces thereof, first and last.

HEART INFIRMITIES, TO CURE.

To put away all Venome from the Heart.

Take Bole Ammoniack, Sanguis Draconis [dragon's blood], of each 3 ounces, of the best Cinnamon 4 ounces; bring them severally by themselves into fine Powder, then mix them well, and take thereof at a time as much as will lie on a six pence, in a cup of Canary Wine, and it will do it.

Against Heart-burning; or the heat in the Mouth of the Stomach.

Take Twenty corns of Oat-meal, and eat them raw; it helpeth; Or, Take 5 or 6 corns of Pepper going to Bed, chew them a little, and swallow them, it doth the like.

Against the beating of the Heart.

Take the Waters of Borage, Bugloss, and Balm, of each a like quantity, and put to them as much Oil of Vitriol, as will make them like Verjuice,[87] and drink thereof first & last a spoonful at a time, and this will heal, tho' of a long continuance.

Another for the same.

Take a pottle of the best Claret Wine, and put therein Baum and Borage, of each one handful, 6 tops of Rosemary, English Saffron 1 drachm, of the best fine Sugar 4 ounces; mingle them well together, then put them into a close Vessel, well stopped, and let it stand by the space of Twenty-Four Hours, then

---

87. *OED* defines as a juice of sour grapes, sour apples, or other sour fruit; from Middle English *verjus*, Old French *vertjus* (verd—unripe).

drink thee of a good draught first and last for Seven or 8 days together, or more, and you shall be helped thereby.

This is Excellent.

To strengthen a fainting Heart, and a weak Stomach.
Take Conserve of red Roses, and eat as much as a Nutmeg at a time, Morning and Evening, is a very great Cordial.

For Fatness about the Heart.
Take the Juice of Fennel and Honey, of each alike, boil them till they be hard, then eat thereof first & last, and be whole.

Good at any time when you are ill.
Take Brandy one ounce and half, Carduus Water one ounce, Sugar-candy powdered one drachm, Saffron one grain, Mace 3 grains; mix them and drink it up.

HÆMORHOIDS.

A Plaster for the Hæmorhoids.
Take Bole Ammoniack, Frankincense; Aloes, Mastick, of each half an ounce, Dragon's Blood three Drachms & a half; powder them all, then mingle them well, and with the white of an Egg beaten and the Juice of Plantain, make them into a Plaster.

A Plaster for the Piles.
Take Dyachylon [white lead] and Oil of Spike,[88] of each a little quantity, melt them in a Saucer, and when they are well incorporated, spread it on a Linnen Cloth, and lay it on the Piles warm, Morning and Evening, and in 4 dayes he shall be whole.

88. Probably oil of spikenard, *Inula Conyza* (ploughman's spikenard) and considered "a good wound herb" by "the older herbalists," according to Grieve, *A Modern Herbal,* 2:760. *Inula* is naturalized in America from Europe.

A Suppository for the Hæmorhoids.

Take Aloes powdered, then mingle it well with Honey, make a Suppository, put it up into the Body, and keep it for long as you can; use this Two or Three times, and be whole.

Another.

And good also for the Fig in the Fundament [hemorrhoids].

Take the Yolk of an Egg, Oil of Roses one ounce, beat them well together, then add white Sugar-candy, and fine Sugar Powdered, Half an Ounce, Saffron in Powder two Scruples, apply it to the Fundament Plaster-wise, and if the pain be more inward, make a Pessary [medicated vaginal suppository], and put it up.

Against the Hæmorhoids.

Take Oil of Eggs, it is a notable Remedy.

HICKET, OR YELKING [LOUD HICCUPS?].[89]

For the Hicket.

Stop both your Ears with your fingers, and the Hicket will presently leave you.

Against the Hicket.

Take the Decoction of Organdy [?], boiled with a few Cloves, and dulcified with a little Sugar, and drink thereof, it helpeth exceedingly. And so olso it provokes Urine, & opens the stoppings of the Liver, Spleen, & Womb.

To Stay the Hicket.

Take Dill, boil the tops thereof in Wine; then tie some of it in a Linnen Cloth, & only smell to it, & it ceaseth.

---

89. Despite the more innovative approaches suggested here, Culpeper recommends only mint in his herbal (*Complete Herbal,* 166).

HOARSENESS, AND LOSS OF SPEECH.

Speech lost, to restore.
Take the Juice of Sage, and the juice of Primrose, of each alike, boil them in white Wine, and gargle it in the mouth.

For a Hoarseness in the Throat.
Take Penny-rial and seethe it in running Water, then strain it, and at Night take a dishful sweetened with a little Sugar, & in 3 times be whole.

Hoarseness, lost Speech, and all Diseases of the Chest and Lungs, to Cure.
Take the Herbs and Flowers of Hedge Mustard, boil them in Wine or Ale, & drink of the Decoction strain'd for a little time. Those by this have been recovered, who have utterly lost their Speech, and almost their Spirits also.

HEALTH TO PRESERVE.

How to provide in hot Countries.
When you travel into Hot Countries, you must observe that Diet which is prescribed in a Fever, that is, not to over eat themselves; use the Juice of Lemons, Rice, white Wine mixed with Endive-water and Vinegar, Cyder, Raisins, Currants, sugar'd Water, & such fresh Meats (moderately) as may be had. Avoid drinking of Sack, Aqua-vitæ, and other hot Drinks, except under the Æquinoctial, or where the Nights are cold; and to provide Oil rather than Butter, and not to be unprovided of Treacle, that is very good.

How to provide in cold Countries.
Those which Sail into cold Countries may feed more liberally, and drink hot drinks safely, because the circundant Air is colder, and so it driveth the heat into the inward parts of the Body, where it fortifies the virtue of Concoction, and helpeth Nature to digest as liberally as it were Winter. I commend unto them also, the use of Tobacco with Oil of Anniseeds (provided they be not of too hot a temper that take it.) And I could wish Seamen to Balast their Ships

with Turneps in Sand, and therein they will be preserved, for Turneps are passing good against the Scurvy, and will defend the Body from such Diseases, as the brackish Air and Diet engender.

ITCH AND SCABS.

A Purge for the inward Cause.
Take first Confectio Hamech[90] 1 ounce, dissolve it in half a Porringer of white Wine over the Fire in the Morning, and drink it fasting. This Purge will take away the inward cause, and purge the Blood.

Against the Itch.
Then take Oil of Roses half a pint, Flower of Brimstone 4 ounces, Mercurius Sublimate 6 grains, Camphore half a Scruple; labour them well together in a marble or in a stone Mortar, and anoint the Body therewith Morning and Evening.

To heal all Itches and Scabs.
Take Plantain-water, Rose-water of each half a pint, of Mercurius Sublimate 2 drachms, crude Allom drachms, powder what is to be powdered, then mix them and boil them in a double Vessel at a soft Fire, for the space of an Hour, then filter it, and use it.

To kill the Itch.
Take one ounce of crude Mercury, boil it in two quarts of Spring-water, till one pint be consumed, then seperate the Quicksilver from the Water, then scratch open the Scabs, and wash them with this Water, and be whole.

To Cure all Scabs, Itch, Tetters, Ringworms, Shingles, and running Sores in any parts of the Body.

---

90. A purging electuary similar to diacatholicon, described by Estes as "a complex cathartic panacea based on cassia and senna" (*Dictionary of Protopharmacology,* 61).

Take four ounces of Plantain Water, 8 ounces of the Brine of Powdered Beef; then boil them together, and scum it clear; then open the Sores, & bathe with this Water, & rub it in well with your Hand. This Cures. *Prob.*

Issues [literally, flows] to make.

Fontanells.[91]

Take Rye-flower and Mustard seed, of each alike, beat them well together to a fine Powder, and with Water make some of it into a Paste; then lay a Ring made of a Rush [genus *Juncus,* often used in baskets or woven wreaths] and lay it on the place where you will have your Issue, there fill the Ring with Paste, and bind it on.

Jaundies [jaundice] Black and Yellow.

For the yellow Jaundies most Excellent, in great Extremity.

Take English saffron two penny worth, of Turmerick and Mace, of each the same quantity, beat them all into fine powder, together, with an indifferent quantity of Rheubarb in Powder, then mingle all with as much fine Sugar as will please your taste, and first and last eat thereof as much as 3 Nuts in the pap of an Apple [i.e., an applesauce consistency].

For the Jaundies.

Take fumitory,[92] and wormwood of each one handful, boil them in Posset-drink or Whey, and being strained, drink of it four ounces first and last.

---

91. From the Latin *Fontana,* meaning "spring" or "fountain." Although it most often refers to the soft spots on an infant's skull (see William S. Haubrich, *Medical Meanings: A Glossary of Word Origins,* 2nd ed. (Philadelphia: American College of Physicians, 2003), 90), the usage here refers to a now-obsolete medical term defined in the *OED* as: "An artificial ulcer or a natural issue for the discharge of humours from the body."

92. Leaves of *Fumaria officinalis.* Considered a tonic for the bowels as well as diuretic, cathartic, diaphoretic, antiscorbutic, emmenagogue, anthelmintic, and a blood purifier. Estes, *Dictionary of Protopharmacology,* 86. Culpeper ascribed all kinds of healing properties to this "tender sappy herb" (*Complete Herbal,* 113–14).

Another for the yellow Jaundies.

Take one drachm of the Seeds of Columbines,[93] finely powdered, and drink it in Wine with a little Saffron in Powder, the same, and sweat two Hours, this opens all Obstructions of the Liver also.

For the same.

Take Southernwood half a handful, white Wine three pints, boil it to a third, and drink thereof six days together.

For the black Jaundies.

Take Earth-worms, slit them and wash them well in white Wine, then so dry them that you may beat them to powder, whereof a Spoonful taken in any Liquor in the Morning Fasting, in a little time it Cureth.

For the Jaundies a quick Cure.

Take Plantain water one Pint, ivory in Powder 2 drachms, Saffron enough to make it yellow, boil them two walms, then strain it, and drink first and last Four Ounces at each time.

KING'S EVIL.[94]

Ointment for the King's Evil.

Take Oil of Bays (not adulterated with Hog's-grease) eight Ounces, Oli-

---

93. Also known as Culverwort, *Aquilegia vulgaris*. Used as an astringent. Grieve, *A Modern Herbal*, 1:214.

94. Most likely an early term for scrofula or cervical lymphadenopathy or tuberculous adentis. However, it might also refer to jaundice since it was also known as *morbus regius*, from the belief that the malady could be cured by the laying on of royal hands. The practice was well known to Culpeper and his contemporaries. The herbalist Parliamentarian's old royal enemy's son, Charles II, who was living in poverty in Paris at Culpeper's death in 1654, assumed the throne six years later and is said to have laid his hands on a hundred thousand afflicted souls in a public relations gesture designed to ingratiate himself with the people. Haubrich, *Medical Meanings*, 127.

banum, Mastick, Gum-Ariback [Arabic], Rosin of the Fir-tree three Ounces of each: distil them, afterwards distil them again with Pot-ashes, and anoint the part.

A Drink for the Evil.

Take white Archangel[95] one good handful, two quarts of Conduit Water, one ounce of sweet Fennel seed, half an ounce of Liquorish clean scraped, boil them to the consumption of half, then let it cool, and being setled, take the clearest, and mix it with two Ounces of Honey of Roses, then make three Draughts first and last.

To Dress the Outward Sores of the Evil.

Take a quantity of Verjuice and fresh Butter, dissolve the Butter in the Verjuice, and wash the Sores well, then lay on the Leaden Plaister (specified in the Title Plaster in this Book) wash them well Morning and Evening.

A Balsom against the Evil Outwardly.

Take half a pint of distilled hot Worm-wood water, put it in a double Glass Bottle of a pint, set it over a few small Cole in a Chafing-dish, and when it begins to warm, put to it half an ounce of the best Myrrh finely powdered, then let it boil a pretty while, then put to it one Ounce and half of Mel Rosatum [rose honey], then let it boil one quarter of an hour more, then take it off, and when it leaves boiling, it is enough.

First, With Linnen Cloaths wipe well the Sores, till they be very dry, then take some Lint, and dip it into the Balsom being Blood warm, and bind them on the Sores twice a day; & use this Diet-Drink following.

A Diet Drink to Cure the King's-Evil.

Take Agrimony, Betony, Liverwort, Self-heal, Comfrey, Bramble Tops, Cardu-

---

95. Also known as white dead-nettle ("dead" because it cannot sting), *Lamium album,* or bee nettle, is a favorite haunt of these honey producers eager for its nectar. Grieve, *A Modern Herbal,* 2:579–80. See also Culpeper, *Complete Herbal,* 15.

us [water?], Wild Tansie, Daisey Leaves and Roots, Plantain Leaves & Roots, Scabious, Sunicle [?], Maiden-hair [*Galium verum* or perhaps maidenhair fern, *Adiantum pedatum*], Mouse-ear [*Hieracium Pilosella*], Poypodium [a fern], and Hempseed, half a handful of each boil them in a Gallon of Water to the consumption of a third part; then put to it three pints of white Wine, then boil them one quarter of an hour, then strain it and put it into the fame Vessel again, with two ounces of the best Senna, Rheubarb half an ounce, four drachms of Jallop, and six ounces of Honey, and let them boil a walm or two, then stop the Pipkin close and lute it, and let it infuse all night over a few Embers; the next day (being cold) strain it & keep it in Bottles; Drink a Wine Glass full in the morning & fast 2 hours after it; then drink a little Broth or Posset-drink clear.

If it be sower before spent, boil it three or four walms with a little more Honey, and having first well washed the Bottle, put in your Drink into the same again. This purgeth out all the Evil Humours in the Body; and the Balsom aforesaid, and this Diet Drink, will absolutely cure Strumæ [scrofula or goiter], i.e., the King's Evil, as hath been often proved.

For the Evil.
Take English Tobacco, stamp it and apply it Plaster wayes to the grieved part it helpeth it in 9 or 10 days very Effectually.

LOOSNESS AND COSTIVENESS.

A Clyster against a Loosness, a present Remedy.
Take three Spoonfuls of Starch made of Wheat; take half a pint of new Milk from the Cow, stir them together, warm them a little and put it up.

To make the Costive loose.
Take a Chicken, and one ounce & a half of new drawn Cassta [perhaps castor, a powerful laxative], boil them together in Fair Running Water, and drink the Broth thereof, and it will make the soluble without Pain.

Against a Loosness.

Take Cinnamon, and Mastich both in fine Powder, of each two drachms, Conserve of red Roses two ounces, mix them well together into a Body, & take thereof the quantity of a nutmeg first and last.

To stop a Loosness.

Take Red Wine and running Water, of each one quart, Cinnamon one Ounce; boil these together to the Consumption of half; dulcifie it a little, and take at a time thereof six Spoonfuls first and last.

LIVER AND LUNGS INFIRMITIES.

Against the Pain of the Liver.

Take Oil of Roses Four Ounces, Rhaponticum in Powder,[96] half an Ounce, of Wax what is sufficient make thereof a Plaster, which you may apply hot to the Grief.

Against the Obstructions of the Liver and Spleen.

Take Eldern Flowers [flower of the elder tree], and Distil them in Balneo Mariæ, of which Water drink three Ounces at a time first and last and you shall see an Excellent success.

Liver and Blood to Cool.

Take the Leaves and Roots of Strawberries, boil them in Wine and Water, of each much alike, then strain it and dulcifie it, which being drunk Four Ounces at a time first and last cools the Liver and the Blood, and assuageth all Inflamations in the Reins and Bladder.

---

96. Monk's rhubarb, *Rheum rhaponticum,* a cathartic. Estes, *Dictionary of Protopharmacology,* 164; Culpeper, *Complete Herbal,* 221.

A Restorative for the Liver and the Lungs, if they were rotten.

Take Fennel roots and Parsley roots, one handful of each; peal away their Bark, take out their Pith, then mince them small, and put them into a Brass Pot to three quarts of Water and boil them; then take Twelve Figs, cut them small and pound them well to the bruising of their Seeds, then put in the Figs together, with a quantity of Honey and Sorrel stamped, and let them boil a while, then take it from the Fire, clarifie it through a Cloth into a Glass and stop it close, that there be no vent, and let the Party drink Four Ounces cold first, and hot last.

To Cure the Ulcers of the Lungs, and to stop Distillations.

Take the Roots of Great Comfrey, boil them in Water or Wine, and take Four Ounces first and last.

To Cure the Imposthumation [a festering or abscess] of the Lungs.

Take Chamomile Water, the Dose is One Ounce first & last. And Fennel Water doth the like.

F i n i s

Appendix

The Simples of *The English Physician*

ALTHOUGH *The English Physician* contains numerous complex and sometimes extremely complicated polypharmacy concoctions, it is not devoid of simples. The following list contains all those preparations involving single-item botanical items (excluding suspension media, flavoring agents, and other excipients) for assorted ailments. These, along with numerous other plants used in combination, would have likely been grown in the family garden and kept on hand in the home. An asterisk denotes plants introduced, naturalized, or adventive from Europe. Of the thirty-two plants listed, seventeen are European transplants.

Agrimony—poison stings and bites

Aloe—hemorrhoids

Black hellebore—fistula

Centaury—poison stings and bites

*Comfrey—"ulcers" of the lungs

Cucumber—red face

*Dill—hiccups

*English ivy, oil of—cramps and flatus

*Fennel—eye trouble (cataracts); juice of—"fatness" of the heart

*Germander—fever

Juniper berries—stomach cramps and diuretic

*Lily (some species naturalized)—burns and scalds; baldness

Marigold—a cordial

*Marjoram—shortness of breath

*Marshmallow—bee stings

Myrrh—bad breath

Pennyroyal (a very similar plant, *Hedeoma pulegioides,* is native to America)—
hoarseness

Peony—convulsions

*Plantain (common plantain, *Plantago major,* introduced from Europe)—
stomach complaints

Poppy (*Papaver somiferum,* introduced from Europe via Turkey and the Far
East)—induces sleep

*Purslain, juice of—rectal bleeding

Rhubarb—bruises

*Rue, oil of—cramps

*Sage, juice of (some species adventive or naturalized from Europe)—bleed-
ing and casting of blood in a consumption

*Southernwood (*Artemesia arboratanum* is the most common)—jaundice

*St. John's wort—spitting and vomiting of blood; to expel blood or choler out
of the stomach

*Strawberry leaves (though there are close cousins native to America, *Fragaria
vesca* was chiefly introduced from Europe)—blood, liver, kidneys

*Thyme—cough

Tobacco —cough

*Valerian (some species native, but *Valeriana officinalis* was introduced and naturalized from Europe)—poor eyesight

Walnuts—fever

Wood betony—shortness of breath, cough, and wheezing

Bibliographic Essay

Reformation Literature, Body and Soul

While the historical milieu of *The English Physician* has been established, it remains to place the work more fully within its proper bibliographic and historiographic contexts. This essay outlines the place of Culpeper's work against the backdrop of appropriate collateral works and considers its role within the tradition of English herbal literature. Its rise from obscurity to become a significant work of early Americana can be seen in tracing its increasing recognition in the secondary literature and as a consequence its citation in the standard reference sources of medical history.

In the introduction we located Nicholas Culpeper within the reformist tradition of the fourteenth-century cleric John Wycliffe. This is in contrast to many later botanic practitioners who often associated their movement not only with Culpeper but also with a different Reformation leader, Martin Luther. As compelling as the link with the Wittenberg rebel may be, there is a disturbingly facile quality to it. For one thing, Luther was German and set his challenge to papal authority within that context. For another, there is nothing in his famous Ninety-five Theses of 1517 (widely available on the Web: for example, Project Wittenberg, Walther Library, Concordia Theological Seminary, http://www.iclnet.org/pub/resources/text/wittenberg/luther/web/ninetyfive.html) that emphasizes the need for Scripture in the vernacular of the people, though Luther did publish a German translation of the New Testament in 1522.

In distinction, Wycliffe was, like Culpeper, a thoroughgoing Englishman. His challenge to authority was multifaceted but chiefly presented through various editions of the English Bibles his Lollard followers issued between 1382 and 1409, predating Luther's effort by well over a century. Both Culpeper and Wycliffe did the unthinkable: they translated (or caused to be translated, in Wycliffe's case) the authoritative texts of their disciplines into English; for Culpeper it was the *Pharmacopoeia Londinensis,* for Wycliffe it was Holy Scripture. The most important version of the Lollard Bibles is available in *The Wycliffe New Testament (1388),* ed. W. R. Cooper (London: British Library, 2002). Cooper's brief but informative introduction is also useful in placing Wycliffe in historical context. Also helpful are: Jonathan Hill, *The History of Christian Thought* (Downers Grove, IL: Intervarsity, 2003); and Christopher de Hamel, *The Book: A History of the Bible* (London: Phaidon, 2001). The latter book includes an entire chapter on English Wycliffite Bibles and presents a detailed history of their development and impact.

The Herbal Literature, 1597–1710

Culpeper's was not the only herbal available to seventeenth-century England. Until his *English Physitian* (1652) burst on the scene, the most famous herbal in England was John Gerard's *The Herball or General Historie of Plantes* (1597), or simply Gerard's *Herbal.* Gerard's flawed (it was a rather imprecise translation of Rembert Dodoen's *Stirpium historiæ Pemptades* [1583] commenced by the late Dr. Priest) but impressive work overshadowed all its predecessors. There is a parallel in Gerard's work with Culpeper's in that many of the remedies found in the earlier herbal appear to be homely cures for common use. Moreover, like Culpeper, Gerard was immensely popular. William T. Stearn has showered Gerard's compendium with praise, calling it "the best-known and most often quoted herbal in the English language" (*Dictionary of Scientific Biography,* 1981 ed., s.v. "Gerard, John").

Hyperbole notwithstanding, it is easy to make too much of Gerard's contribution, a fact that becomes clearer once more important dissimilarities with Culpeper are examined. In contrast to the feisty but unconnected Culpeper, Gerard was no stranger to the rich and powerful. In 1577 he managed the gardens of William Cecil, Queen Elizabeth's chief minister and closest confidant.

Also unlike Culpeper, who was a complete outsider from the medical establishment, Gerard was very active in London's Barber-Surgeon Company and in 1608 he rose from junior warden to master of that recognized guild. In fact, Gerard was well known to the medical elite, having served as curator of the College of Physicians' physic garden from 1586 to 1604, and it was probably through that association that he originally came into possession of college physician Robert Priest's *Stirpium* manuscript.

Not only were Culpeper and Gerard men standing on very different rungs of the social ladder, but they also produced very different works. Gerard's *Herbal* work was massive, containing nearly fourteen hundred pages and over two thousand woodcuts, making this a comparatively expensive volume. This kept it from reaching the broader audience of Culpeper's more modestly composed and priced titles. Interestingly, royalist Thomas Johnson produced a lavishly illustrated edition of Gerard's *Herbal* in 1633 that purported to "compete" with Culpeper, but again, its expense kept it out of the hands of the very masses that could have elevated the name of Gerard to equal that of his nonconformist counterpart. For all Gerard's importance as a contributor to the English herbal tradition, it was Culpeper's style that made him truly unique; his irreverent jabs at the medical establishment and its wealthy patrons was unlike anything witnessed before. More than just an author of domestic medical guides, Culpeper spoke the language of the people both literally and figuratively. Booksellers of the day knew this translated into sales and profits. William London listed no fewer than fourteen Culpeper titles in his famous *A Catalogue of the Most Vendible Books in England* (London: self-published, 1658).

Thus, several reasons can be offered to explain why Gerard's work never reached the popularity or stirred up the controversy of Culpeper's herbal. First, Gerard's *Herbal* was not as widely distributed to the general public as were Culpeper's works; second, Gerard's *Herbal* did not come infused with the same lively style and invective as did Culpeper's titles; third, the authors were themselves associated with the medical establishment very differently (Gerard as someone still within the pale; Culpeper as a dangerous outsider);

and fourth, perhaps most significantly for our purposes here, Gerard never came close to Culpeper's impact upon America. As pointed out in the introduction, Patricia Watson's seminal work on preacher-physicians in colonial New England (see the section on secondary sources on p. 105) indicates that Culpeper's works were the most widely used of all medical texts; out of nineteen medical authors surveyed, Gerard did not even make the list.

Next to Gerard, the most important English herbal during this period was John Parkinson's *Theatrum botanicum.* Its publication in 1640 made it the largest catalog of botanicals to date, comprising some thirty-eight hundred plants. Like Gerard, Parkinson filled his book with woodcuts. He also adorned his title page with the stylized figures of Adam and Solomon, representing labor and wisdom. Despite its impressive size, no amount of labor or wisdom could raise it above Gerard's or Culpeper's herbals. Although Parkinson's work is considered by some to be finer than Gerard's, his imposing title probably caused many to shy away in preference to what appeared to be the more readable Gerard volume.

Perhaps more closely parallel to the work in hand is *The Skilful Physician.* Written by the pseudonymous Dr. Deodate and published in 1656, it appeared seven years after Culpeper's *Physical Directory* and four years after his *English Physitian.* For those interested in an easily accessible, well-informed text essentially contemporary with Culpeper (it appeared just two years after his death), *The Skilful Physician,* edited by Carey Balaban, Jonathon Erlen, and Richard Siderits (Amsterdam: Harwood Academic, 1997) is strongly recommended. The editors not only provide a useful introduction, offering some interesting comparisons with Culpeper's *English Physitian;* they also add helpful commentary for all the preparations found therein.

As discussed earlier, Culpeper was so popular that all kinds of titles were attributed to him. Copycat printers eager to garner sales produced a mind-boggling array of materia medicas, guides, vade mecums, handbooks, herbals, dispensatories, and directories bearing the name if not the genuine content of the author. Nevertheless, the English herbal tradition produced one author who honestly followed Culpeper's style and approach but still produced a genuinely new work: William Salmon and his *Botanologia: The English Herbal or History of Plants* (London: I. Dawkes, for H. Rhodes, 1710). Next to Culpeper's, Salmon's herbal was the most popular work of its kind in the American colonies.

But Salmon's herbal marked the end of an era. By the eighteenth century the literature was turning from mere lists of plants and recipes to more complex domestic health guides. More narrative and broader-ranging domestic medical books allowed for more detailed and diverse health advice than their herbal counterparts. It was in the tradition of the minister as healer that John Wesley produced his well-received and much-used *Primitive Physick, or, An Easy and Natural Method of Curing Most Diseases* (London: Thomas Tyre, 1747). Similarly, William Buchan's *Domestic Medicine, or, The Family Physician,* first published in Edinburgh by Balfour, Auld, and Smellie in 1769, appeared in numerous editions throughout the remainder of the century and into the next. These became models for American productions, the most important of which was Samuel Thomson's *New Guide to Health, or, Botanic Family Physician* (Boston: E. G. House, 1822). Sometimes authors put a distinctly American spin on their work, as when Peter Smith titled his medical guide *The Indian Doctor's Dispensatory, Being Father Smith's Advice Respecting Diseases and Their Cure* (Cincinnati: Browne & Looker, 1812; repr. *Bulletin of the Lloyd Library,* no. 2, Reproduction Series, no. 2 [1901]). Yet all of them traced their lineage to those works in the herbal tradition that helped bring medicine to the masses—the most widely distributed of which were those of Nicholas Culpeper.

A Bibliographic Context for *The English Physician* (1708)

Presenting a coherent bibliographic context for this edition of *The English Physician* is complicated by the problem of attribution. The fact that the book is really a reprinting of *Physical Receipts, or, The New English Physician* (1690), issued in London by Thomas Howkins, has been noted earlier. But we know little of Howkins. Apparently he flourished during the last two decades of the seventeenth century. His chief interests appear to have been in alchemical, materia medica, and sundry scientific texts. For example, in 1685 he printed and sold *Four Books of Johann Seger Weidenfeld, Concerning the Secrets of the Adepts; or, of the Use of Lully's Spirit of Wine. A Practical Work . . . Collected out of the Ancient as Well as Modern Fathers of Adept Philosophy* and *The First Book of Menstruums.* The following year he issued from his press *Clavis horologigæ; or, A Key to the Whole Art of Arithmetical Dyalling . . . Whereunto is Annexed an Appendix, being the Explication of the Pyramidical Dyal Set Up in His Majesties Garden at White-Hall, 1669.* He produced a *Catalog of Friends Books* in 1687, of which only a fragment has survived. The same year he produced the *Physical Receipts* he also published (with a John Harris) *The Treasury of Drugs Unlock'd, or, A Full and True Description of all Sorts of Drugs, and Chymical Preparations, Sold by Drugists.* He was also involved in publishing (again with John Harris) *Medicina practica, or, Practical Physick. Shewing the Method of Curing the Most Usual Diseases Happening to Humane Bodies* in 1692. His extant productions would suggest he was a busy compiler and repackager of medical titles, making his *Physical Receipts* in keeping with the extant corpus of his work.

That said, his *Physical Receipts* is only nominally more the result of the printer's ingenuity than of Culpeper's pen. It is clear that Howkins compiled this from a variety of sources, the exact nature of which are now buried with this once-busy publisher. Some passages *are* lifted straight from Culpeper; others, however, are modifications of his remedies; still others bear no relationship to anything known to have come from Culpeper. At any rate, the book would have nearly disappeared altogether had it not reappeared on the other side of the Atlantic under a new title from the ambitious and innovative press of Mr. Boone. Since those details have already been discussed at length, they need not be recounted here.

Nevertheless, there is another difficulty besides spurious authorship with *The English Physician,* namely, the struggle of Culpeper's publications to gain standing within the medical literature. Much of this is undoubtedly due to the persistent tinge of quackery surrounding the herbalist. The single most important arbiter in the field is *Morton's Medical Bibliography,* often referred to by its earlier title, *Garrison and Morton's Medical Bibliography*. *Garrison and Morton* has been slow to recognize Culpeper as a legitimate writer of noteworthy medical literature. From its first edition in 1943 through its fourth in 1983, there was no mention of Culpeper in its pages. Interestingly, in its fifth edition (Brookfield, VT: Gower, 1991), *Garrison and Morton* finally included Culpeper among its entries, and even *more* interestingly, both are American productions: entry 1828.1 is the present volume reprinted here, listed as "the first medical book (94 pp.) printed in North America;" and entry 1828.2, his *Pharmacopoeia Londinensis; or the London Dispensatory*, issued in 1720, is listed as "the first *full length* [emphasis added] medical book published in North America."

Like *Garrison and Morton*, the authoritative *Medical Books, Libraries, and Collectors* by John L. Thornton (now titled *Thornton's Medical Books*) has been slow to recognize Culpeper. There was no mention of him at all in the first edition in 1949. Only in the 1966 edition did Thornton allot about two pages to the contributions of this "keen classical scholar" who was, in Thornton's words, "probably no worse than most of the physicians of his period" (London: Andre Deutsch, 103). In the third edition the editor, Alain Besson, gave Culpeper slightly more coverage (Brookfield, VT: Gower, 1990, 69, 91, 96, 104–6). This belated recognition has been a direct result of the secondary historical literature, which has increasingly revised its view of the much-maligned herbalist.

Secondary Sources

For nearly 250 years Boone's production remained hidden away in the dusty recesses of a few rare book rooms in the United States. Although James F. Ballard, appointed director of the Boston Library in 1928, was probably the first to appreciate it as the first medical book published in British North America, it was David L. Cowen's "The Boston Editions of Nicholas Culpeper," *Journal of the History of Medicine & Allied Sciences* 11 (April 1956): 156–65, that really presented *The English Physician* to the scholarly community. The work of resurrecting the career of Culpeper himself began with F. N. L. Poynter, librarian at the renowned Wellcome Medical Library of London. His two articles, "Nicholas Culpeper and His Books," *Journal of the History of Medicine & Allied Sciences* 17 (January 1962): 152–67 and "Nicholas Culpeper and the Paracelsians," in *Science, Medicine, and Society in the Renaissance: Essays to Honor Walter Pagel,* ed. Allen G. Debus (New York: Science History, 1972), 1:201–20, did much to recast the herbalist of Spitalfields in a more sympathetic light. Instead of curtly dismissing Culpeper as a quack and poseur, Poynter saw him as a champion for a more populist medicine and an informed critic of the questionable materia medica of his day.

More recently, Culpeper has been the subject of book-length biographies. First is Olav Thulesius, *Nicholas Culpeper: English Physician and Astrologer* (New York: St. Martin's, 1992). Although he treats Culpeper sympathetically, the author has the disconcerting habit of filling in details without supporting evidence. Although Thulesius's biography has much useful information and should be read carefully by any student of Culpeper, caution is in order: conversations are included that seem probable but lack primary documentation, and certain passages seem to have more literary flair than historical precision. Significantly better is Benjamin Woolley's *Heal Thyself: Nicholas Culpeper and the Seventeenth-Century Struggle to Bring Medicine to the People* (New York: HarperCollins, 2004). In a book twice the length of the Thulesius biography, Woolley also paints a positive portrait of his subject and offers considerably more *documented* details concerning Culpeper's life and times.

Biographical particulars aside, Culpeper's publication record is full of unexpected twists and turns, enough to unsettle the most diligent student. It seems nothing is simple when it comes to the Culpeper bibliography; everything from attribution to edition to publisher is full of mischief and intrigue. A real help in sorting through these difficulties is Mary Rhinelander McCarl's "Publishing the Works of Nicholas Culpeper, Astrological Herbalist and Translator of Latin Medical Works in Seventeenth-Century London," *Canadian Bulletin of Medical History* 13 (1996): 225–76. Although her thesis that Culpeper was a merely doing the bidding of his printers seems strained and unwarranted, McCarl's essay shows meticulous research and includes important information on attribution, edition, and publisher details related to the corpus of Culpeper's work not readily available elsewhere. In short, it is an unparalleled one-stop bibliographic guide to Culpeper.

As crucial as Culpeper is in understanding and contextualizing *The English Physician,* Nicholas Boone is to some extent even more important. Had it not been for George Emery Littlefield's *Early Boston Booksellers, 1642–1711* (1900; repr., New York: Burt Franklin, 1969), hours—indeed days or weeks—of tedious record combing in New England repositories would have been necessary to reconstruct the life of this early American printer. As it is, Littlefield presents not only considerable biographical data on Boone but also offers a thorough account of the printing trade in colonial Boston. Littlefield's book was indispensable in the writing of my introduction.

As mentioned earlier, Culpeper had an appreciable impact upon the botanical sectarians of nineteenth- and early-twentieth-century America. Information and influences in that regard can be found among the leaders and partisans of the movement, such as Wooster Beach, *American Practice of Medicine and Family Physician,* 10th ed. (New York: James McAlister, 1847); Alexander Wilder, *History of Medicine* (Augusta, ME: Maine Farmer, 1904; and John Uri Lloyd, *Origin and History of All the Pharmacopeial Vegetable Drugs* (Cincinnati: Caxton, 1929). Additional material is available in John S. Haller Jr.'s *The Medical Protestants: The Eclectics in American Medicine, 1825–1939* (Carbondale: Southern Illinois University Press, 1994) and his *The People's Doctors: Samuel Thomson and the American Botanical Movement, 1790–1860* (Carbondale: Southern Illinois University Press, 2000). For discussion on the movement as a whole, see Alex Berman and Michael A. Flannery's *America's Botanico-Medical Movements: Vox Populi* (New York: Pharmaceutical Products, 2001).

Finally, there are a number of sources that helped the navigation through the complex fields of colonial American studies, therapeutics, and pharmacy to locate more accurately Culpeper's place and importance in medical culture and *The English Physician*'s place in history and literature. Several studies were particularly helpful in understanding medicine and health care in the New England colonies: George E. Gifford, "Botanic Remedies in Colonial Massachusetts," in *Medicine in Colonial Massachusetts, 1620–1820* (Boston: Colonial Society of Massachusetts, 1980); J. Worth Estes, "Therapeutic Practice in Colonial New England," also in *Medicine in Colonial Massachusetts;* Patricia A. Watson, *The Angelical Conjunction: The Preacher-Physicians of Colonial New England* (Knoxville: University of Tennessee Press, 1991); and George B. Griffenhagen and James Harvey Young, "Old English Patent Medicines in America," *Pharmacy in History* 34 (1992): 200–28. Useful in placing Culpeper within the broader context of English herbal literature was Eleanour Sinclair Rhode's classic monograph, *The Old English Herbals* (1922; repr., New York: Dover, 1971); J. Worth Estes, "'To the Courteous and Well Willing Readers': Herbals and Their Audiences," *Watermark* 18, no. 3 (1995): 63–70; and Barbara Griggs, *Green Pharmacy: The History and Evolution of Western Herbal Medicine,* 2nd ed. (Rochester, VT: Healing Arts Press, 1997). Also critical in establishing Culpeper's work within the larger framework of pharmaceutical history were the following: Charles H. LaWall, *Four Thousand Years of Pharmacy: An Outline History of Pharmacy and Its Allied Sciences* (Philadelphia: J. B. Lippincott, 1927); James Harvey Young, *The Toadstool Millionaires* (Princeton, NJ: Princeton University Press, 1961); David L. Cowen, *The Colonial and Revolutionary Heritage of Pharmacy in America* (Trenton: New Jersey Pharmaceutical Association; and Madison, WI: American Institute of the History of Pharmacy, 1976); and Glenn Sonnedecker, *Kremers and Urdang's History of Pharmacy,* 4th ed. (1976; repr., Madison, WI: American Institute of the History of Pharmacy, 1986).

Sources Informing the Main Text

Having covered the sources for the introduction, it remains to discuss those bearing upon *The English Physician* reprinted here. Perhaps the most interesting and important one is the reference to a genuine Culpeper title, the so-called *Complete Herbal.* This work has a complex history all its own. It should be noted that some permutation of Culpeper's "herbal" (originally *The English Physitian*) has been in continual print since it first appeared in 1652, and various editions abound. One year later Culpeper put out a second edition. By the 1800s publishers like London's Virtue & Company were combining *The English Physitian* with Culpeper's *London Dispensatory* (his 1653 translation of the second *Pharmacopoeia Londinensis,* not to be confused with his earlier *Physical Directory,* which was his translation of the first pharmacopoeia of 1618) and calling it, rather disingenuously, *The Complete Herbal.* So, in effect, this long-lived but bastardized title is really a combination of two Culpeper works. These industrious reprinters took certain other liberties with the work: for example, placing "M.D." after Culpeper's name (something not found in his contemporaneous publications), changing "Physitian" in the title to "Physician," and so on. But by and large, in their main sections these versions remain faithful renderings of the original texts.

The commemorative tercentennial edition issued in Birmingham, England, is the one selected here. The first 290 pages consist of Culpeper's alphabetized herbal, pages 281 to 361 contain assorted directions and lists of roots, barks, woods, herbs, flowers, fruits, seeds, and grains; "tears, liquors, and rosins"; juices; "things bred from plants"; living creatures; "parts of living creatures and excrements"; things from the sea; and "metals, minerals, and stones." On page 362 Culpeper's irreverent but insightful and sometimes humorous commentary on the *London Pharmacopoeia* begins and continues to page 553. This is all that can be confidently ascribed to Culpeper. Beginning on page 554 are several additions (*not* used in contextualizing the present work), starting with "A Key to Galen's Method of Physic," then continuing on page 584 with "Culpeper's Last Legacies: Select Medicinal Aphorisms and Receipts for Many Diseases Our Frail Natures are Incident To," an allusion to a posthumous publication titled *Culpeper's Last Legacy,* discussed in the introduction but bearing little resemblance to the original. At the very end are sixteen color plates of various herbs which, because of their expense to produce, never appeared in any of Culpeper's original works.

It is worth noting that the particular copy of Culpeper's *Complete Herbal*

Index